Do You Want to Look Good Naked?

*Natural Weight Loss
in 6 Easy Steps*

**DAVID DESJARDINS
& HELENE DUMAIS**

Published by Transit Publishing Inc.

ISBN: 978-1-926745-27-5

Cover design: François Turgeon
Text design and composition: Arnaud Oddon
Interior drawings: Dany Dubé

Cover photo:
© Stockbroker

Transit Publishing Inc.
1996 St-Joseph Boulevard East
Montreal, QC
H2H 1E3

Tel: 514-273-0123
www.transitpublishing.com

Printed and Bound in U.S.A.

Thank You Dany and Marie-Julie...

For an open mind, early on, toward a project that may have seemed,at times, doubtful to ever see the light of day.

For being patient as we spent countless hours at a computer. Dany, for your generous time and effort with your illustrations...for being patient with us and regularly adapting your work to our everchanging minds...for your ideas and your suggestions.

Marie-Julie, for your remarkable generosity with editing and translating contributions...your relentless research and review lectures... your trial recipes...your ideas and suggestions...if this book was our child, you'd surely be its godmother.

Thanks also to both for all those things you did that had nothing to do with the book but that enabled us to focus on the project at hand. And especially, Dany and Marie-Julie, thank you for your love and friendship.

With much gratitude

I am a young 58 retired police/security officer who is so grateful to David and Helene for their support in helping me get healthier and feel better about who I am. For most of my life I had been extremely active and in great health. As time went by the pressures of my job, lack of attention, knee surgery and recoup times all left their toll. At 56 I was an unhealthy 308 pounds. I am 6'4 and thought I could carry it well but then came the day. The day was when I saw pictures of myself with friends at a dinner party. I took a double take because the person I saw in the pictures was not me. Yes, smiling and happy but so overweight and looking uncomfortable. With a grandson on the way I decided I had to do something. David and Helene came into the picture. With care and attention they provided me with a "new way of eating" (I refuse to call it a diet), that actually worked wonders. I was actually shocked how quickly things changed from the first week. I immediately started to feel better and see amazing results. Now at 228, I feel great; the lost weight helped my knee and other health issues. From the compliments I have been getting, I also look great. The best part is that this "new way of eating" works for me. So easy in fact that I no longer even think about it. I just enjoy my food... including my steak!!

I was very lucky. I was lucky to reach out to people who love their food and love life. They provided very clear easy methods to readjust my eating habits. They provided me with the continued support to make good eating a habit and not a chore. Yes initially you have to make an effort but the results are instantaneous and will encourage you to press forward.

Enjoy their book and be religious in following its advice. You will be amazed every day you will look in the mirror, dressed or naked!!

M.J. Bialek
Former Bodyguard to World Leaders

CONTENTS

Part 1

By David

"Better to live one year as a tiger, than a hundred as a sheep."
– Madonna

FAQ

"What is this book about?"

This book contains a weight loss program for individuals who are REALLY ready to do something about those
extra pounds.

It's not about selling you something.
It's not about helping you find the motivation to be in action.
It's not about introducing you to yet another weight loss program that yields no results.

No. It's much more than that.

If you know the extra weight has been in the way of your sexiness, your beauty and your drive, then this book is for you.

Technically, our weight loss program gives you new tools and guidelines on healthy eating, exercise, rest, sleep and stress management. *Experientially*, however...well, just imagine how life would be today if those extra pounds were gone...forever...

That's what this book is about.

"I've tried a lot of weight loss programs and diets...how is this one better?"

Most weight loss programs and diets are created inside of popular social paradigms (Calorie counting, RDAs, good fats VS bad fats, Food Pyramid, eating according to blood types, etc.), which are, in turn, created out of economic interests...and this is why they fail.

Most people gain and regain more weight with each attempt at dieting—also known as the "yo-yo syndrome." Our program is different because it is designed to respect our biological heritage (i.e., the way we were meant to operate physiologically according to Mother Nature) and, consequently, produces *healthy*, *balanced*, *safe* and *sustainable* results.

"Is this program good at any age? Maybe I'm too old to lose weight?"

Our program is good for people of all ages. Its success is not age dependent. The beauty of this program is that, by giving you guidelines adaptable to your goals and to your lifestyle, you are always in complete control of the weight loss experience. It was designed to be very adaptable and to keep in mind various factors; for example, we are very aware that a guideline stipulating "vigorous" exercise will be adapted differently by women than by men, by young than by old, by sedentary than by active, etc.

No one is too young or too old to lose weight and look good naked.

"I suffer from an illness...can I still do this program?"

It is your constitutional right to prescribe for yourself. We do recommend, however, that, ill or not, you consult with your physician before taking on any lifestyle changes. Our method is designed for weight loss, not curing disease.

Please note that the body cleansing process induced by our weight loss program may cause discomforts along the way. These may occur, and if they do, are usually mild and temporary (e.g., mild headaches, mild skin eruptions, and changes in feces). As the extra pounds disappear, a feeling of energy and overall well-being is created, quickly making any temporary discomforts a thing of the past.

"Is this scientifically proven?"

If by "scientifically proven" you mean "endorsed by the government or by medical experts", well, parts of our program are and parts of our program aren't. We have taken the best of what traditional and alternative medicines have to offer and, most importantly, we have perfected it over the years through trial and error by designing weight loss programs for individuals at large. We value experience and long-term repeatedly proven results over any "official" expert opinion, and it is the fruit of these successful experiences that we share in this book.

"Will it take long to get the results?"

We would love to be able to predict with precision "how much" and "by when", but given the many individual differences influencing weight loss, this is not possible. Some factors are not within your control (like gender, age, past eating and exercise habits), while others are (like how much weight you aim to lose and how motivated you are at integrating the program), and it's by focusing on the latter that you'll be able to better guess "how much" and "by when".

Just to give you an idea, some of our clients have lost as little as 1 pound per week, while others have lost as many as 8 (even at this rate, everything was done safely and healthily...).

"Will I need to make drastic changes to my lifestyle?"

Because "drastic" has such a relative meaning, the answer to this question really depends on your definition of the word. How we perceive steps necessary in obtaining a desired result is usually shaped by the certainty we have of getting this result. In other words, if you were 100% certain to lose weight by doing this program, very few lifestyle changes would appear as "drastic" because your motivation would make you unstoppable in the face of any challenges or obstacles. Helene and I know our program works, and we know how amazing it feels to be slim and fit, therefore we do not consider any lifestyle changes contained herein as "drastic".

If you are reading this book, it's because your lifestyle hasn't given you the results you desire, so you will need to make changes. Like anything new, these lifestyle changes *may* seem drastic at first, awkward, confusing, hard and downright illogical...but they also *may not*. It all really depends on who you are and, at this point, it's only by trying it that you'll find out.

Life Before This Book

You are physically attractive.

You are sexy.

You like to bite into life. You work hard and you play hard, and this enables you to succeed both professionally and socially.

As a result, you are very self-confident.

...as long as you have clothes on...

...because the moment you have to get naked, down to your "undies" or in a bathing suit, the walk-tall-&-proud person that you are suddenly feels uneasy and begins mentally listing all the reasons justifying why your body is the way it is...

"It's genetics."

"I don't have time to exercise as much as I would like to."

"In my line of work, it's impossible to eat healthy!"

"The day I'm really ready, I will do something about it..."

"Compared to others, I'm not half bad!"

Sounds familiar?

As far as we're concerned, you either have *results*, or the *reasons* why you don't have these results. Unless one suffers from an illness, with a little effort, anyone can lose weight. No excuses. This book is much like a treasure map, the pot of gold being weight loss, of course.

We've designed an easy to follow step-by-step program, keeping physiological explanations to a minimum in order not to supersize the book's contents. Also, contrary to popular trend, we have included very few references from "credible" weight loss sources, scientific documents, medical journals and health experts' opinions, knowing full well that, given the right price, any "expert" will and has published "hard scientific data" proving just about anything.

In the words of Timothy Ferriss, from his book *The 4-Hour Workweek*:

"...expert status can be created in less than four weeks if you understand basic credibility indicators and what people are conditioned to equate with proof of superior knowledge."

"It is possible to know all there is to know about a subject—medicine, for example—but if you don't have M.D. at the end of your name, few will listen. The M.D. is what I term a "credibility indicator." The so-called expert with the most credibility indicators is the one who will sell the most product, not the one with the most knowledge of a topic."

"The commonsense rules of the "real world" are a fragile collection of socially reinforced illusions."

Real experts are the ones who have done it, who have proven results, and not some individual with any more than a nice diploma on his office wall. It's OK to accept information from others, but this information should *always* go through your common sense and instinct filters first (not to be confused with your "conditioned" filters).

Presently, you may only have *a few* pounds to lose, or you may have *many*. Either way, our 6-Step Weight Loss Program will yield your desired results. In this book, you will discover a new lifestyle where you don't have to count calories, you don't have to focus on low fat this or sugarless that, where exercise can actually be fun and where managing weight is entirely within your control!

Because we live in a weight-promoting world, integrating our program will be challenging at first but, as you get the hang of it, will become easier. Whatever challenges come your way, just remember *why you are doing what you are doing* and, throughout, *don't forget to have fun!*

David & Helene
January 17th, 2009

P.S. *Looking Good Naked* is an accomplishment on its own; one of the many other perks, of course, is how good you'll feel with your clothes on...

The Program

"People avoid change until the pain of remaining the same is greater than the pain of changing."

– Anthony Robbins
best-selling author, keynote speaker, motivational coach and
advisor to World leaders

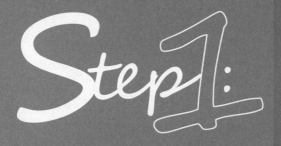

Step 1: Understanding Those Extra Pounds

"Beautiful young people are accidents of nature, but beautiful old people are works of art."

– Eleanor Roosevelt

"I have all these great genes, but they're recessive. That's the problem here."

– Calvin
of *Calvin & Hobbes Comic Books*

Today's most accepted weight gain theory[1] states that increased fat storage occurs when a person takes in more calories than the body needs or uses.

We have a slightly different theory.

We do not believe that what gets stored up in your fat tissue is simply a surplus of calories, but rather a surplus of *toxins*.

Calorie: fuel or energy value of a food.
Toxin: a substance the body cannot use at a given moment.

We also believe that the body, when unable to eliminate a surplus of toxins, sets these toxins aside in tissues where they will be least harmful (in most cases fat tissue) until it can eliminate them through its proper channels (e.g., sweat, urine and feces). *If toxins accumulate, weight gain occurs.*

---

1 - This does not include "intentional" weight gain, as is the case with some athletes (e.g., boxers, wrestlers and body builders) or weight gain due to a metabolic disorder (e.g., trauma or tumors in the food-regulating centers of the brain, endocrine diseases such as Cushing syndrome or hypothyroidism, heart or lung disorders).

There are 2 types of toxins:

1. **The ones we take in from our environment**, i.e., air and water pollutants, chemicals we put on our body (e.g., make-up, sun protection lotions and moisturizing creams), and unusable substances in food.

2. **The ones produced from the many chemical reactions occurring inside our body**, i.e., carbon dioxide, urea, uric acid, lactic acid, creatine, creatinine, bilirubin, ammonium salts, undigested parts of food, inorganic salts, products of bacterial decomposition, excess vitamins (from supplements, especially fat-soluble A, E, D and K), calcium oxalate, calcium phosphate crystals, ketone bodies and urobilinogen.

The human body has built-in mechanisms for toxin elimination (e.g., bowels, lymphatic system, lungs and kidneys), but when these mechanisms are overtaxed, toxins accumulate and weight gain occurs.

Supporters of the common calorie theory often end up confused and frustrated. They watch what they eat and count their calories, yet still gain weight. They burn off a substantial amount of calories through regular exercise, yet do not lose sufficient weight. With our theory, you'll modify specific lifestyle components so that toxins do not accumulate, thus losing weight by:

- **Reducing the quantity of toxins coming into the body,**

  especially by transforming your dietary, as outlined in Step 3. Although some toxins may enter the body by way of skin and lungs, these do not have an impact on weight gain nearly as important as that of food, which is why we'll focus on the latter.

- **Reducing the quantity of toxins created inside the body,**

  especially by changing your lifestyle as it pertains to food, sleep and stress management; these lifestyle elements are elaborated respectively in Steps 3, 5 and 6.

- **Increasing the amount of toxins being expelled from the body,** especially by integrating healthier exercise and sleep patterns, as outlined in Steps 4 and 5.

Understanding those extra pounds is that simple. Weight gain and weight loss needn't be confusing ever again.

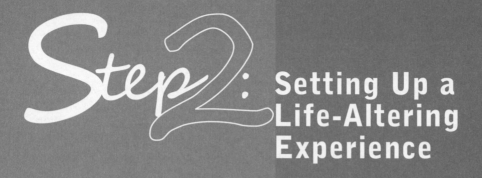

Step 2: Setting Up a Life-Altering Experience

"Preparation, I have often said, is rightly two-thirds of any venture."

– Amelia Earhart
first woman to fly across the Atlantic and set a number of records for "firsts" for women as a pioneer aviator

"If you really want something, you can figure out how to make it happen."

– Cher

Most diets and weight loss programs are very short-lived. Quick results may be acheived, but then something happens and usually the weight returns, often more than before... and this, even if you continue to apply their concepts and guidelines!

Our program is different.

Transform your lifestyle according to the contents of this book, and you will obtain your desired weight loss results...guaranteed. Maintain this new lifestyle, and you will never have extra weight ever again... ever. Do the program until you reach your goal and then go back to your present lifestyle, however, and the weight will come back... also guaranteed.

It is important to know that, as soon as you begin to apply the concepts and guidelines contained in the 6 steps of the program, you will also begin a 3-part linear experience:

Your Starting Point ➔ Your Transition Period ➔ Your Results

Your Starting Point

> *"The starting point of all achievement is desire."*
> **– Napoleon Hill**
> best-selling author of *Think and Grow Rich*

Your starting point is defined in part by your body's *toxicity level*, this being the amount of toxins present in your body at any given moment. The greater the toxicity level as you begin your weight loss program, the more work your waste management faculties will have in eliminating these toxins, so the longer it will take to lose weight.

Your starting point is also defined by your body's *metabolic state*. This is your body's ability to perform its physical and chemical processes, by which material substances are produced, maintained, and destroyed, and by which energy is made available. Here are a few examples to illustrate the various components of the metabolic state:

- An athlete's cells will burn sugar at a different rate than someone who has never exercised.
- A person living in cold Nordic weather will have different body temperature-regulating capacities than an individual living in a warm tropical climate.
- Someone living at sea level will use up oxygen differently than someone living in high mountainous altitudes.
- An individual having had a dietary high in junk food will use up nutrients from food today differently than a person having had a dietary low in junk food.

In other words, the lifestyle habits and activities you have had thus far in life have conditioned your body to conduct its physical and chemical operations differently than someone who has had different lifestyle habits and activities. Hence, two individuals participating in the same weight loss program will react differently because of different metabolic states.

If, over the years, you have conditioned your body to be a fast-paced, high-energy and well-oiled machine, then you will start this weight loss program with a metabolism that is in a state to conduct toxin elimination very rapidly and efficiently. Past factors contributing to a finely tuned metabolic state are, for example:

- good stress management
- healthy eating habits
- regular exercise
- proper rest and sleep
- healthy stimulation and motivation
- limited use of drugs (prescribed or recreational) and alcohol

The less your body has been conditioned by these lifestyle factors, the less efficient your toxin elimination will be. *It does not mean your body will not be able to eliminate ANY toxins; it simply means that it may take a little longer for you to lose weight and that the symptoms of transition may be different than would those of someone with a very healthy past.*

The starting point of your weight loss program can be compared to the starting point of a waste management crew. The bigger the heap of garbage (toxicity level), the more work for the crew, and the longer it will take to get the job done. On the other hand, a more experienced crew (metabolic state) will get the job done faster and more efficiently.

Setting up a Life-Altering Experience

Your Transition Period

"Not everything that is faced can be changed, but nothing can be changed until it is faced."

– Lucille Ball
American comedian and star of *I Love Lucy*

The Wedding Dress

Because she lived overseas, Johanna hadn't seen her family for over 6 months. The wedding was in 2 weeks. A few years ago, when she had gotten engaged, her mother had offered her wedding dress, passed down from her own mother. Johanna had been thrilled at the idea of getting married in the same church and with the same dress as both her mother's and grandmother's... thrill that ended about a year after the engagement, however, for Johanna had gained weight... the dress would fit no more. From that point on, even though her mother never said anything, there had always been a silent uneasiness every time wedding conversations came up. Her mother had still inquired, maybe once, as a mother would, about her plans to get a new wedding dress; Johanna had been able to keep her in the dark, saying there had been delays and it would only be ready last minute.

And now, she was driving up to her parents' house. For the last week, Johanna had imagined the look on their faces, playing it over and over in her mind, as she would step out of the car and they would see that she had lost the weight...

She knew her mother would cry.

Once you start the program, you need to be aware that your body will be in a transition period between *your starting point* and *your results*. During this period, you will have *symptoms of transition*. These symptoms are a result of your body having suddenly more energy to conduct its cleaning and repair functions. In other words, create a new lifestyle in which you eat healthier, exercise more, sleep better and manage stress more efficiently, and the resulting extra energy enables the body to expel stored up toxins.

The types of symptoms you get depend a great deal on your starting point (toxicity level + metabolic state). These will also depend on how much rigor you bring to the program. Going "cold turkey" means stronger transitional symptoms, but quicker results. Doing it more gradually, on the other hand, equals milder symptoms, but slower results. While transitional symptoms may vary from one individual to the next, here are some common ones:

- light-headedness
- headaches (with variable intensity)
- skin eruptions (mild acne-like)
- changes in feces/urine (smell, color, consistency, frequency)
- light to mild weakness in legs during sustained effort (e.g., while going up stairs)
- changes in sleep quantity and quality (body craving more sleep initially, but then needing less sleep over time)
- increased mucus production (runny nose, expectorations)

It is important to understand that these symptoms are nothing but toxins being eliminated from the body. Please do not panic. Don't go thinking: "*I feel worse since I started this weight loss program...I now have symptoms I never used to have before...I should discontinue this immediately.*" These symptoms are a mere reflection of the body's cleansing process and are, in a way, a necessary evil. You should not look to suppress them with drugs, cure-like concoctions or any type of home remedy. Let the body run its toxin elimination process unhindered.

Granted, when such symptoms appear, it is not a common reflex to simply leave them be. We get headaches, we take pills. We cough and sniffle, we take syrup. We get skin eruptions, we use cream. As you go through the 6 steps of the weight loss program, your body will begin to cleanse itself. Do not interfere or else you will only impair this toxin elimination. Remind yourself that what is occurring is for a greater cause (i.e., reducing your weight and consequently being healthier). Know also that these symptoms are temporary...which brings us to *duration*.

As you may have guessed, the *duration* of your transition period is somewhat unpredictable, since it depends on characteristics unique to you (i.e., your toxicity level, your metabolic state, your rigor and your discipline). It is difficult to designate arbitrarily what constitutes adequate duration for this transition because of the unique nature of individual characteristics.

In regards to *speed*, however, be assured that the body will conduct its toxin elimination process at the healthiest of speeds. That's the beauty of our program: because it is based on the physiological laws that govern metabolism, the body will take off just the right amount of weight at just the right pace. Be patient and trust the body's innate wisdom.

Just like a New Year's resolution, motivation for the program may start off strong and be fueled by good intentions, but this motivation may also quickly wane. *Because motivation is the key ingredient to the success of your weight loss program, anticipate how you are going to maintain this motivation, should it begin to fade.* Install failsafe mechanisms so as to prevent laziness and past conditioning from taking over. It is important to set up the context to ensure success. In order to do this, use the following questionnaire:

Knowing myself, what are some of the highly probable (not certain, but probable) reasons why my weight loss program may go astray? *Example*: I hate doing anything that feels like discipline.

- _____

- _____

What can I put in place so that little red warning flags come up if these probable failure causes start to creep in?

Example: The moment I begin to curse and complain about my weight loss program, I need to be in communication with my best friend to tell him/her (and to remind myself...) why I chose to do this program in the first place.

- _____

- _____

What solutions can I think of before any of the warning signs even show up?

Example: Make a promise to my best friend that, if and when times get tough, I will be in communication (e.g., a phone call) immediately to get some support.

- _____

- _____

Your Results

"Excellence is not a singular act, but a habit. You are what you repeatedly do."

– Shaquille O'Neal
NBA MVP and 4 times NBA Champion

*O*btaining *weight loss results* and *maintaining these results* are very different experiences. *Weight loss* is usually easier because it is much shorter in duration (weeks/months VS a lifetime) and, like any new project, motivation is strong at the beginning. *Weight control*, on the other hand, is and will always be a constant challenge because of society's weight-promoting nature. Here are a few suggestions to help with weight control:

• **Until You Get the Hang of It, Always Carry This Book with You.**

You will notice from the information in Step 3 that most meals in today's society are weight-promoting. Consequently, we suggest that, until you've memorized this information, you have this book handy, because the better you are at *identifying* healthy foods/meals, the easier it will be to keep weight off.

• **Exercise Regularly.**

This may sound cliché, but it is important to be in action because we all know that there are tons of good excuses NOT to exercise. Local gyms and neighborhood asphalt are not always the most motivating places for physical activity, before or after a hard day's work. Exercise will be discussed further in Step 4.

• **Know That People Around You May Try to Discourage You in Your New Weight Loss and Weight Control Lifestyle.**

Most individuals do not like change, and they much prefer that the people around them (this being you) stay just as they have always been. Even worse, others may be jealous and may not want you to look like a million bucks, afraid of having a living shining health specimen too close to them as a constant reminder

Setting up a Life-Altering Experience

of how overweight/unhealthy they really are...sad, but true. Once you start losing weight, you may have to deal with other people's opinions and remarks. True friends will be happy for you, and will greet you with *"Wow! You look fantastic!"*, while others will be who they always are, and be quick with the *"Is something wrong? Are you sick? You are losing too much weight. Be careful, you will become too skinny."*

Chances are you may even become a social black sheep (a good looking sexy black sheep mind you, but a black sheep nonetheless); nothing that'll get you fired or burned at the stake, of course, but enough that you find it annoying, so just be prepared.

- **Establish Your Own "Looking Good" References.**

You will find yourself cross-referencing your new look with social standards. Vogues and fashions are created out of economic interests, and not always with your health in mind. Stay away from "what you should look like" according to magazines, billboard ads and TV; instead, aim to transform your body to simply feel good and sexy... according to your own personal preferences

- **Know That Dealing with Temptation to Indulge in Weight-Promoting Foods Will Become Easier.**

In the short-term, dealing with temptation will be solely a question of determination...either you'll give in, or you won't. In the long-term, however, we have noticed that the healthier you are and the more balanced is your lifestyle, the less temptation occurs. A healthier body has fewer cravings for unhealthy foods and weight-promoting activities.

Moreover, the more balanced are your daily/weekly stimulations, the less you will be tempted to deviate. For example, if most of your weekly hours are spent on monotonous things like commuting, working and doing house chores, then you need to balance them out with fun, play and leisure. If you don't, you will be looking for quick fixes under the form of rewarding junk food, comforting TV time, relaxing alcohol or mood altering drugs. Managing stress and re-structuring your schedule will be discussed further in Step 6.

- **Know That Maintaining a Healthy Weight Is a Condition Obtained from What You Do As a Rule, and Not As an Exception.**

Even up to this day, after years of being very healthy, Helene and I still eat things like chocolate, ice cream, burgers and fries...and we also sometimes feel lazy and skip a few planned exercise sessions... which also means, consequently, that we get poorer sleep. So even we, weight loss and weight control "gurus," occasionally give in to the weight-promoting demons of this world but, in order to stay on track, always use the following 80/20 guideline: *at least 80% of our lifestyle is non weight-promoting, while no more than 20% is allowed for "cheat" moments.*

If you are going to use the "80% rule and 20% exception" guideline, beware of a common trap: *how it appears to be may not be at all how it really is.* Rare are the individuals who keep a detailed journal of their weekly eating, exercise and sleeping habits and, when asked if they were good this week, are *convinced* they were. We have seen this many times with our clients: they were certain they were following the 80/20 guideline, yet, much to their incomprehension, were not getting their anticipated weight loss results; we would then ask them to keep a weekly journal detailing food, exercise and sleep, and it was only then that they realized the disparity between *their impression* and *the reality* of what was going on.

So, if you are not fulfilling on your desired weight loss results, start keeping a journal and get the true facts. As soon as you experience dissatisfaction with weight loss or weight control, let that be a warning sign.

On a last note to Step 2, be sure to re-think your agenda for upcoming weeks, in regards to social activities that could jeopardize the success of your program: restaurant outings, birthday parties, drinking fests, etc. Let friends and family know that you may not accept *all* invitations, and that you may even politely decline some meal offerings; don't forget to also make room for ample sleep time, for your body's elimination faculties will greatly appreciate it. By preparing the next few weeks this way, you give yourself a chance to build a strong weight loss foundation; once it's in place, dealing with weight-promoting temptations will be much easier.

Now, one last issue remains: *Do you really want this? Are you REALLY ready to change your life?* Contrary to diet shakes, fat burning pills or liposuction, our program requires effort. As you will learn, however, it's more than just a weight loss experience...it's a very healthy way to live.

OK. Enough said. Time to say goodbye to that extra weight, one last time...

Mirror Drill and Dream List

"Please God, if you can't make me thin, make my friends fat!"
– Unknown

The Mirror Drill is very simple: stand naked in front of a full-length mirror, and look at your body from all angles. Take as much time as you see fit. Get close, stand back some, take in all views. Make sure you take a good long look at some of what you'll never see again.

Next, create a Dream List by identifying all motivational outcomes related to weight loss. Eating better and exercising more are not very motivating things by themselves. What is motivating, however, is what these lifestyle changes make possible, like having your curves admired at the beach, getting compliments from co-workers, getting that sexy dress you've been meaning to buy, finding a mate, etc. Visualize your future at a time when the weight is off, dream a little, and this will give you the necessary motivation for the program.

Program Set-Up Checklist

Simply insert "yes," "no," "N/A" (for "not applicable") or a time & date in the appropriate cells.

	Done	Not done yet, but will be done by... (insert time & date, then make a promise to a friend that it will be done by established time & date, and then call him/her when it's done)
Have I put failsafe mechanisms in place to ensure motivation?		
Have I clearly established my own references for "looking good"?		
Have I created a journal that will permit me to apply the 80/20 guideline?		
Have I re-arranged my schedule in order not to have too many weight-promoting temptations in the next few weeks?		
Am I really ready to do this weight loss program?		
Did I do the Mirror Drill and create my Dream List?		

Step 3: Relearning How to Eat

"If we all worked on the assumption that what is accepted as true were really true, there would be little hope of advance."

– Orville Wright,
(along with brother Wilbur) inventor of the world's first successful airplane

"Who was the first guy that looked at a cow and said, "I think that I'll drink whatever comes out of those things when I squeeze them?"

– Calvin,
of *Calvin & Hobbes Comic Books*

There are many schools of thought as to what constitutes "healthy eating" but, unfortunately, most of them produce weight gain. There are probably just as many schools of thought on weight loss...and while some may produce the desired weight reduction, these results are usually:

- Unsafe (e.g., weight loss occurring too rapidly)
- Unbalanced (e.g., high-protein diet)
- Short-lived (e.g., soon after the weight loss results, more weight than before suddenly appears, often referred to as the "yo-yo syndrome")

You may think those extra pounds you are carrying are not due to your eating habits, but they are. You may, in fact, be *convinced* you eat quite healthily and that the extra weight does not come from food, but you are mistaken. Your conditioning and beliefs are strong. There is no other reality than the one you presently know about food. If you are serious about shedding weight, however, then you need a new reality, so here it is.

The problem with popular food guidelines and weight loss diets is that they do not take into account 2 very important concepts:

1. **In order for proper digestion to occur, certain chemical compatibilities (i.e., food combinations) must be respected**; these are elaborated throughout this chapter.

2. **In order for nutrients to be used by the body, they must be in a state that is *bioavailable*.** This is the extent to which a nutrient can be absorbed and used by the body; for example, iron in a spoon is not *bioavailable* to the human body, while iron in a peach is. If our system cannot use parts of food, these become toxic.

If improper digestion occurs or if ingested nutrients are of a non-bioavailable nature, toxins accumulate and weight gain is produced.

If you want to lose weight, you will have to re-learn how to eat and factor in these 2 very important concepts. If you do not, you will *inevitably* gain weight. There is no other way, for weight management is a function of our physiological design as humans, and not what "experts" say or what trends dictate.

In order to take into account these essential concepts, we have created the following Recommended Eating Guidelines. As you read on, keep in mind that these Guidelines are not designed to *only* work if you apply them 100%. If you can assimilate and integrate them to your lifestyle fully overnight, then great, but because you have conditioned yourself to eat a certain way *your whole life*, we expect their application to take some time. In the beginning, you will obtain weight loss results even with just *partial* application; the more you integrate these Guidelines into your new lifestyle, however, the more results will occur.

You will also find a checklist and charts immediately following this chapter to help summarize its contents; use these daily, post them on your fridge and make copies to leave in your car and at work, for they were designed to facilitate your new process of relearning how to eat.

Recommended Eating Guidelines:

1. Respect gastric evacuation times.
2. Do not eat proteins and fats/oils at same meal.
3. Do not eat proteins and starchy foods at same meal.
4. Do not eat proteins and sweet foods at same meal.
5. Do not eat starchy foods and acid foods at same meal.
6. Do not eat fruits with any other type of food.
7. Eat melons only with other melons, nothing else.
8. Do not eat sweet fruits with acid fruits.
9. Simplify your meals.
10. Avoid drinking with your meals.
11. Reduce your intake of refined foods.
12. Reduce your intake of non-foods.
13. Reduce your intake of animal products.
14. Reduce your intake of irritants.
15. Reduce your intake of cooked foods.
16. Do not overeat.
17. Do not eat when tired.
18. Do not go to sleep with food in your stomach.

You will notice that eating according to these Guidelines makes life a little more complicated...well, in fact, *quite a bit* more complicated.

We wish it wasn't so.

We wish you could keep eating like the "experts" tell you and not ever have to worry about gaining weight ever again.

But that isn't so either.

At this juncture in your life, you will have to choose whether you are ready or not to *re-learn how to eat*. It may be awkward at first, but the good news is that eating in order to promote weight loss and to prevent any additional weight from ever occurring again is possible... and it can be savory, fun and easy. You just need a little re-training, that's all. If you're ready to make the jump, then please, read on.

GUIDELINE NO.1: Respect Gastric Evacuation Times

Once you swallow food, it travels through your digestive tract in the following manner:

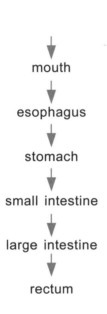

↓
mouth
↓
esophagus
↓
stomach
↓
small intestine
↓
large intestine
↓
rectum

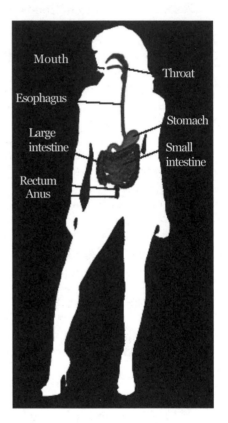

As it travels, nutrients are absorbed into the lymph and blood streams, leaving the non-usable parts to continue and form excrement. Food must be broken down from bigger complex molecules to smaller simpler ones before this absorption can take place. For example, proteins are broken down into amino acids, starches (complex sugars) into simpler sugars and triglycerides (complex fats) into simpler fatty acids.

For this breakdown to occur, food undergoes *mechanical* digestion (i.e., your teeth cut and grind, and the muscles in your stomach and intestines churn) and *chemical* digestion (i.e., digestive juices are secreted in various parts of your digestive tract). If you ate protein *by itself*, say just chicken (no rice, no potatoes, no beverage, no dessert, not even a glass of water!!), it would take approximately 6 hours before it was completely evacuated from your stomach and into the small intestine, where it would undergo final digestion and absorption into the blood and lymph. The evacuation of food from your stomach occurs progressively (small quantities at a time) as a circular muscle (called the pyloric sphincter, which separates your stomach from your small intestine), opens intermittently. This process by which food slowly passes on from your stomach to your small intestine is called gastric evacuation. If you do not allow for proper gastric evacuation to occur, food sits in your stomach and, under high body temperature and bacterial activity, spoils and creates a toxic load.

Please note that gastric evacuation times are **approximations**. Many factors (i.e., age, gender, fatigue, the presence of caffeinated foods, meal size, etc.) can either delay or accelerate this process. As a general rule, the longer you wait, the better the chances of this process occurring properly. Here are different food types, with their approximate gastric evacuation time at the bottom right corner:

PROTEINS

Animal products
Dairy products
Eggs
Fish
Fowl
Meat
Seafood

Plant products
Nuts
Seeds
Soy beans (tofu)
Sprouts

6h

FATS/OILS

Animal fats
Butter
Cream
Etc.

Animal oils
Cod liver oil
Etc.
Avocado

Vegetable oils
Corn oil
Safflower oil
Etc.

4h

STARCHY FOODS

All cereals
Carrots
Lentils
Mature corn
Peanuts
Potatoes
Rice
Sprouted grains
Etc.

Flour-based products
Breads
Crackers
Cakes
Nachos
Cookies
Pasta
Muffins
Etc.

4h

NON-STARCHY VEGETABLES

Alfalfa sprouts	Bok choy	Broccoli	Brussels	Celery
Cauliflower	Celery cabbage	Chayote	sprouts	Eggplant
Kale	Kohlrabi	Lettuce	Cucumber	Rappini
Turnips	Turnip tops	Zucchini	Okra	
			Sweet bell	
			peppers	

Cabbage (young and sweet), Escarole (if not bitter), Green beans (young and tender), Mustard greens (if young and mild), Squash (all summer varieties),

Green corn (if not mature, and if eaten less than 2 hours after picking), Etc.

3H

MELONS

Canary
Cantaloupe
Honeydew
Watermelon
Etc.

45min

SWEET FRUITS

Banana
Date
Dried fruit
Fig
Sweet grape
Etc.

75min

SUB ACID FRUITS

Apricot
Blueberry
Mango
Nectarine
Pear
Sweet apple
Etc.

60min

ACID FRUITS

Grapefruit
Lemon
Orange
Pineapple
Strawberry
Sour apple
Etc.

60min

The following categories have *highly variable* gastric evacuation times because of the wide variety of items or ingredients used in their making:

- The "Refined Sweets" category: refined white sugar, for example, eaten by itself and on an empty stomach, has a gastric evacuation time of less than 30 minutes, whereas ice cream (because of the fat content), more than 1 hour, and cake (because of eggs, flour and all other ingredients), more than 4 hours! *As a practical rule, allow 30 minutes for the simpler items (brown sugar, white sugar, maple syrup, honey, etc.) and up to 4 hours for the more complex items (cake, cookies, fudge, ce cream, etc.).*

REFINED SWEETS

Brown sugar
Cake
Cane syrup
Chocolate
Cookies
Corn syrup
Fudge
Honey
Ice cream
Maple syrup
Milk sugar
Molasses
Muffin
Pie
Raw sugar
Sweeteners
White sugar

All other varieties

30min/4h

- The "Beverages" category: freshly squeezed orange juice, for example, taken by itself and on an empty stomach, leaves the stomach in approximately 30 minutes, but alcohol can stay for hours. *As a practical rule, estimate 1 hour for all items in this category, except alcohol where you may include up to 2 hours.*

BEVERAGES

Healthy	Weight-promoting
Coconut juice	Alcohol
Extracted e.g., carrot juice	Carbonated drinks
Freshly blended	Coffee
Freshly squeezed	Milk
Maple water	Tea & herbal teas
Water	Beverages with additives (sugars, flavors, colors, electrolytes, etc.)
	Processed beverages (pasteurized, from concentrate, boiled, steamed, etc.)
	All other beverages which are not listed

1h/2h

- In the "Acid Foods" category: coffee, for example, stays less than 1 hour (caffeine stimulates gastric evacuation) but vinegar more than 1 hour. *As a practical rule, estimate 1 hour for beverages (coffee, tea, carbonated drinks) and tomatoes, and 3 hours for all other items (vinegar, salad dressings, endives, etc.).*

ACID FOODS

Beet tops	Salad dressings
Bitter cabbage	Spinach
Carbonated drinks	Swiss chard
Coffee	Tea (certain varieties)
Endive	Tomato
Escarole (bitter)	Vinegars
Rhubarb	

1h/3h

In regards to this first Recommended Eating Guideline on gastric evacuation, you may be thinking...

"I have to wait 6 hours after protein before I can eat something else! That's too long!"

"Four hours after muffins to be able to eat an apple, that's crazy!"

Well, I can understand your reaction. You and I and everyone else have been conditioned to eat a certain way for years; unfortunately, this conditioned way of eating leads to weight gain. If popular guidelines such as calorie counting and eating from the Food Pyramid really worked, extra weight wouldn't be such an omnipresent phenomenon. Granted, it's hard not to listen when doctors, health experts and our very own government are giving us guidelines, but then you have to ask yourself: *What's more important, what so-called experts are saying, or obtaining true weigh loss results...?*

There is no escaping our physiological design. Respecting gastric evacuation times is the first step.

Gastric Evacuation Delayed

The gastric evacuation process is slowed or completely suspended during sleep and exercise, thus prolonging times given in this section. For example, if you eat a protein food, wait 1 hour and go to sleep for 8 hours, then your gastric evacuation period is not 9 hours total; during the first hour, some of the protein would get digested but then, because of suspended digestion, bacteria living inside your digestive tract would act on the remaining bulk and putrefaction (rotting) would occur. Please note that it really is guess work at this point, for it is difficult to evaluate gastric evacuation times in such situations. The same applies to exercise: during any activities more intense than walking (e.g., running or swimming), gastric evacuation is usually slowed or suspended.

GUIDELINE NO.2: Do Not Eat Proteins and Fats/Oils at Same Meal

The first steps of protein digestion occur in the stomach and require an acid environment, at a pH of approximately 2. Fats and oils, on the other hand, require a different environment at a pH of 5 to 6. Although both environments are acid in nature, they are sufficiently different to impair one another's activity. Eating proteins and fats/oils at the same meal is thus not recommended. Up until recently, science, its PhDs and its multimillion-dollar machines did not acknowledge the value of food combining. They held that whatever went into the stomach simultaneously got digested. Nutritional concepts are slowly changing and food combining is finally seeing the light of day. Our experience has shown that there are certain chemical incompatibilities that cannot be ignored in the pursuit of adequate weight management. Years of designing successful weight loss programs will attest to this fact. Try it and you will see for yourself.

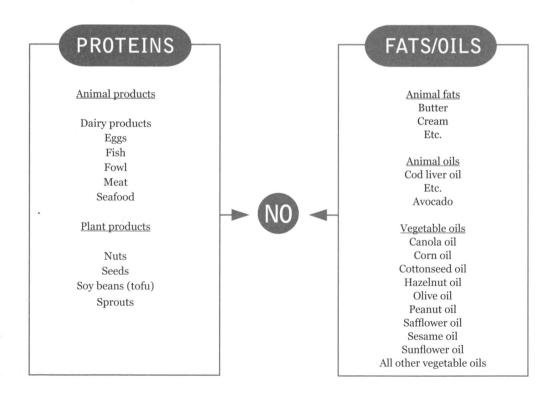

PROTEINS	FATS/OILS
Animal products	Animal fats
	Butter
Dairy products	Cream
Eggs	Etc.
Fish	
Fowl	Animal oils
Meat	Cod liver oil
Seafood	Etc.
	Avocado
Plant products	
	Vegetable oils
Nuts	Canola oil
Seeds	Corn oil
Soy beans (tofu)	Cottonseed oil
Sprouts	Hazelnut oil
	Olive oil
	Peanut oil
	Safflower oil
	Sesame oil
	Sunflower oil
	All other vegetable oils

NO

Fat

It is not because you eat fat that you will get fat... this is a popular myth. If you eat excess fat, then yes, you will gain weight, but this is not unique to fat...if you eat excess anything, be it proteins, sugars, etc., then you will also gain weight. Eating the wrong types of fat—saturated fat, for example—can also promote weight gain.

As you will notice in Part 2, there are many recipes including avocado, cream and/or butter...you may eat these recipes without any worry of gaining weight. Social conditioning regarding fat will kick in and make you hesitate and doubt, but rest assured, you'll still lose weight.

GUIDELINE NO.3: Do Not Eat Proteins and Starchy Foods at Same Meal

As stated previously, protein digestion in the stomach requires an acid environment at a pH of approximately 2. Starchy foods, however, require a much higher pH, anywhere between 6.35 and 7.40 (depending on the sources you consult).

Again, if both a protein and a starchy food are in the stomach together, digestion is impaired and weight gain occurs.

As you will see from the following lists, the combinations of protein and starchy foods constitute most of today's meals, like meat and cheese sandwiches, pasta and meat, pasta and fish, fish and rice, seafood and rice, meat and potatoes, meat and pizza dough, cheese and pizza dough, anything made with a combination of flour-eggs-milk (like cookies, cakes, muffins, breads, etc.). These poor combinations are everywhere, but it's not because they are popular that it makes them any less weight-promoting. In the words of novelist Anatole France, *"If a million people say a foolish thing, it is still a foolish thing."*

PROTEINS

Animal products
Dairy products, e.g., clabber, cheese, cow milk, goat milk, ice cream, yogurt
Eggs, e.g., chicken egg, ostrich egg, guinea fowl egg, fish egg
Fish, e.g., cod, grouper, haddock, halibut, salmon, shark, tuna
Fowl, e.g., chicken, guinea fowl, pheasant
Meat, e.g., beef, deer, horse, lamb, pork
Seafood, e.g., crab, lobster, mussel, oyster, prawn, scallop, shrimp
All other animal parts, e.g., liver, brain, intestine, tongue

Plant products
Nuts, e.g., almonds, cashews, hazelnuts, macadamias, pecans, pine nuts, pistachios
Seeds, e.g., pumpkin, sesame, squash, sunflower
Soy beans (tofu)
Sprouts, e.g., bean, soy, sunflower seed

NO

STARCHY FOODS

All flour-based products
Barley
Beets
Buckwheat oats
Carrots
Chestnuts
Coconuts
Dry beans
Dry peas
Edible pod peas
Globe artichokes
Jerusalem artichokes
Lentils
Lima & other beans in the pod
Mature corn
Mature green beans in the pod
Millet
Oats
Parsnips
Peanuts
Peas in the pod
Potatoes
Pumpkin
Rice
Rutabaga
Rye
Salsify (oyster plant)
Sprouted grains
Water chestnuts
Wheat
Winter squash
Yams & sweet potatoes

Now, this guideline is a biggie for most people...

"Can't have fish with rice...that's nuts!"

"Meat and potatoes don't mix? But I've done it my whole life, and everyone I know is doing it, so it must be OK..."

"Do you realize what this means?! No more pizza, spaghetti, lasagna, hamburgers, ham & cheese sandwiches, steak & baked potatoes, seafood & rice...it's way too restrictive! You've just eliminated more than half of all of today's meals!"

We've heard it all and believe me, Helene and I understand the reaction. We've been there. We had the same reaction when we first began to realize the implications of such an eating guideline, but we've applied it to our own lifestyle and to that of countless others since, and guess what? *It works!* The weight has come off and has never come back and, in the presence of such inspiring results, eating choices become very easy.

But wait, there's more...

GUIDELINE NO.4: Do Not Eat Proteins and Sweet Foods at Same Meal

Protein by itself in the stomach can stay up to 6 hours before having completely moved on to the small intestine. Sweet foods (high in simpler sugars) need to leave the stomach much sooner than that; if they don't, they ferment really quickly.

If you chew both protein and sweet in the same bite, what you swallow is very well mixed together. If you alternate one bite of protein and one bite of sweet stuff, they end up stacked on top of one another and form a pile in the stomach. Either way, because there are no gastric mechanisms to first separate the different types of food, and then hold one off (protein) into the stomach while the other (sweet food) exits at its base and on to the small intestine, sweet foods will be held up with the protein. Under body core temperature (99.86°F or 37.7°C), sweet foods will ferment rapidly, bacterial decomposition will set in, and this will thwart protein digestion.

Furthermore, many acids (as found during protein digestion) tend to destroy sugar molecules. As a result, both protein and sweet food will go to waste, thus increasing the body's toxic load and contributing to weight gain.

This is a hard one for dessert lovers. You can have, say, steak and salad, but then you'll have to wait 6 hours for dessert!

The problem gets compounded if the protein meal is salty (which is often the case when it comes to meat, fish, fowl or cheese preparations) because it'll make you thirsty (not good; see Guideline no.10) or crave something sweet which, when combined with a protein, would only cause more fermentation.

There are no miraculous solutions...either have something other than protein, or have it and wait out the appropriate gastric evacuation time of 6 hours.

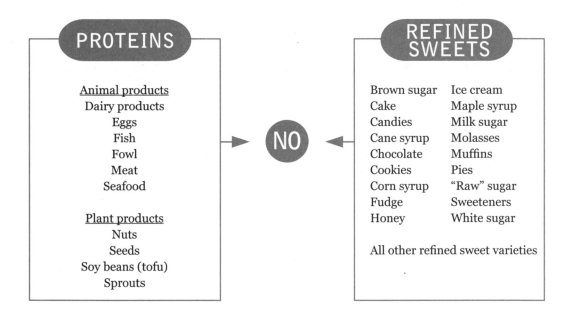

PROTEINS		REFINED SWEETS	
Animal products		Brown sugar	Ice cream
Dairy products		Cake	Maple syrup
Eggs		Candies	Milk sugar
Fish	NO	Cane syrup	Molasses
Fowl		Chocolate	Muffins
Meat		Cookies	Pies
Seafood		Corn syrup	"Raw" sugar
		Fudge	Sweeteners
Plant products		Honey	White sugar
Nuts			
Seeds		All other refined sweet varieties	
Soy beans (tofu)			
Sprouts			

GUIDELINE NO.5: Do Not Eat Starchy Foods & Acid Foods at Same Meal

Starchy foods require a very low acid to slightly alkaline digestive milieu. Many acid foods are so acidic they impair starch digestion. Any impaired digestion promotes weight gain.

Sorry folks...toast and coffee...spaghetti and tomato sauce...fries and ketchup...all out!

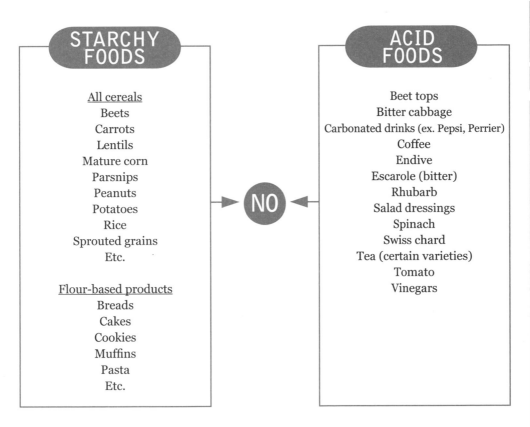

STARCHY FOODS

<u>All cereals</u>
Beets
Carrots
Lentils
Mature corn
Parsnips
Peanuts
Potatoes
Rice
Sprouted grains
Etc.

<u>Flour-based products</u>
Breads
Cakes
Cookies
Muffins
Pasta
Etc.

NO

ACID FOODS

Beet tops
Bitter cabbage
Carbonated drinks (ex. Pepsi, Perrier)
Coffee
Endive
Escarole (bitter)
Rhubarb
Salad dressings
Spinach
Swiss chard
Tea (certain varieties)
Tomato
Vinegars

GUIDELINE NO.6: Do Not Eat Fruits with Any Other Type of Food

Because fruits have a quicker gastric evacuation time than other food types (proteins, fats, starchy foods, vegetables, etc.), it's best to eat them alone. A popular trend is to eat fruits for dessert...this promotes weight gain because fruits are held up longer than they should in the stomach and, under high body temperature, rapidly spoil. On an empty stomach, you may eat fruits 1 hour before a non-fruit meal, but never *with* or *immediately after* such a meal.

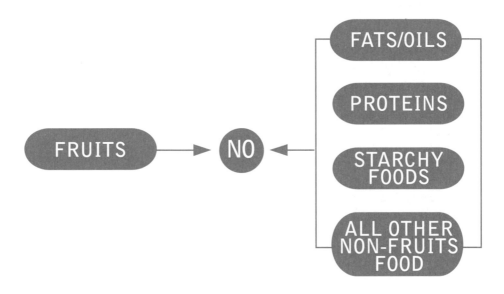

GUIDELINE NO.7: Eat Melons Only with Other Melons, Nothing Else

Melons are the most fragile of all fruits, digestively speaking. Eaten on an empty stomach, melons will stay no longer than 45 minutes in the stomach before moving on to the small intestine. It is therefore OK to mix melons with other melons, but not with any other fruit or any other type of food, as these have longer holding time in the stomach... so no melon cubes in fresh fruit salads, and no melon for dessert.

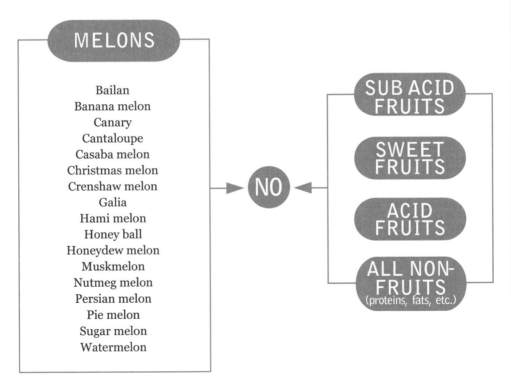

MELONS

Bailan
Banana melon
Canary
Cantaloupe
Casaba melon
Christmas melon
Crenshaw melon
Galia
Hami melon
Honey ball
Honeydew melon
Muskmelon
Nutmeg melon
Persian melon
Pie melon
Sugar melon
Watermelon

NO

SUB ACID FRUITS

SWEET FRUITS

ACID FRUITS

ALL NON-FRUITS
(proteins, fats, etc.)

Science and Human Nutrition

For some reason (economic, most likely...), nutritional science has drawn erroneous conclusions from anatomical and physiological findings over the course of history. For example, research has identified that the human body needs certain vitamins and minerals. Nutritional experts then created vitamin and mineral supplements in the form of pills in order to supply us with these nutrients... a good intention, but something very important was forgotten along the way, *that the human body can only use what is bioavailable.* In other words, vitamin and mineral supplements are in a form not accessible to and not usable by the body, and what is not usable becomes toxic, thus creating an accumulation of toxins that leads to weight gain (amongst other things).

The same goes for digestion: notions like the importance of properly combining meals and the importance of waiting for gastric evacuation before piling up new food into the stomach have not been popularized. Why? Well, take a good look around... who would suffer (economically) if weight problems and digestive problems suddenly disappeared? We're talking HUGE industries here.

The point is this: because science has not spent a lot of time studying proper food combining and important digestive processes like gastric evacuation, we must operate today with what little information we have. Be assured, however, that there is enough information in this book to get you started and going in the right direction. It's based on *millions* of people's experience, as found in literature by such noted health experts and/or best-selling authors as Dr. Sylvester Graham, Dr. Russell Thacker Trall, Florence Nightingale, Mary Grove, Harriet Austin, Susanna May Dodds, Ellen White, Louisa May Alcott, Dr. Herbert M. Shelton, Bernarr Macfadden, Hereward Carrington, Otto Carque, John H. Tilden, Linda Burfield Hazzard, Harvey & Marylin Diamond, John Robbins, Dr. John A. McDougall, Jean Rocand, Ann Wigmore, Dr. Brian Clemens, T.C. Fry, Mike Benton, Dr. Virginia Vetrano, etc... and, most importantly, our experience and that of our clients since 1996.

In addition, you will compile information that is unique to you. For example, we've listed an approximate gastric evacuation time of 4 hours for potatoes... if you're tired when you eat them, it may take longer... if you purée them or eat smaller portions, it may be quicker... you may find that you can cheat more often than you thought and still lose weight... etc. In time, you will try, adapt, adjust and mold a lifestyle that is perfect for your needs.

GUIDELINE NO.8: Do Not Eat Sweet Fruits with Acid Fruits

Sweet fruits possess high-sugar content. Acid fruits, on the other hand, possess both sugars and acids, and these exist in a ratio where the former are not present in sufficient quantities to be destroyed by the latter. A sweet fruit's high-sugar levels coming in contact with an acid fruit's high-acid levels, however, will ruin sugar molecules and consequently increase the toxic load.

SWEET FRUITS	SUB ACID FRUITS	ACID FRUITS
All dried fruit	Apricot	All citrus
Banana	Blackberry	Grapefruit
Date	Blueberry	Lemon
Fresh fig	Cherimoya	Lime
Persimmon	Grape	Orange
Sweet grape	Huckleberry	Pineapple
	Litchi	Pomegranate
	Mango	Sour apple
	Mulberry	Sour cherry
Some sweet fruits are not listed. A predominant sweet taste is a good indication of their classification.	Papaya	Sour grape
	Pear	Sour peach
	Raspberry	Sour plum
	Sweet apple	Strawberry
	Sweet cherry	Tomato
	Sweet nectarine	
	Sweet peach	*Some acid fruits are not listed. A predominant sour taste is a good indication of their classification.*
	Sweet plum	
	All sub acid fruits are not listed. Some may bear the name "sweet," but the taste predomination should be the determining factor... in this case, neither sweet nor sour (a little of both).	

 YES   YES

 NO

The Tomato

Scientifically speaking, the tomato is a fruit...culinary speaking, however, it is considered a vegetable. Digestively speaking, it falls into a category of its own: it is acid, therefore should not be mixed in with starchy or sweet foods, but it also doesn't have the sugar content of acid fruit, and is thus a good mix with protein foods. You will find the tomato in both the "Acid Fruits" and the "Acid Foods" categories of this book.

Please note that there are "regular" and "low acid" tomatoes, but the difference is negligible, so we consider them as one item only.

GUIDELINE NO.9: Simplify Your Meals

Many of today's foods are made up of a plethora of substances, thus increasing chances of chemical incompatibilities. For example, if you had a meal made up of a ham & cheese sandwich, garden salad, glass of milk and chocolate wafer cookies, this is what you would actually be putting into your body (ingredient lists taken from America's leading brands):

Regular white bread: *enriched wheat flour, water, glucose-fructose sugar, vegetable oil, yeast, salt, soybean flour, sodium stearoyl-2-lactylate, monoglycerides, acetylated tartaric acid, esters of mono and diglycerides, calcium propionate, ammonium chloride, calcium iodate.*

Mayonnaise: *soybean oil, water, whole eggs, egg yolks, vinegar, salt, sugar, lemon juice, natural flavors and calcium disodium EDTA.*

Fat-free processed ham: *ham, water, salt, sugar, sodium lactate, sodium phosphates, sodium diacetate, sodium erythorbate, sodium nitrite.*

Fat-free processed cheese: *whey, milk protein concentrate, water, sodium phosphate, dried corn syrup, salt, sodium hydroxide, lactic acid, sodium citrate, milk fat, sorbic acid, artificial color, carrageenan, cellulose gum, artificial flavor, sodium tripolyphosphate, citric acid, calcium phosphate, disodium inosinate, milk, vitamin A plamitate, apocarotenal (color), annatto (color), enzyme, cheese culture.*

Salad: *lettuce, tomatoes, celery.*

Italian dressing: *vinegar, water, soybean and/or canola oil, corn syrup, sugar, salt, spice, monosodium glutamate, onions, garlic, lemon juice concentrate, xanthan gum, potassium sorbate, calcium disodium EDTA, parsley, oleoresin paprika.*

Milk: *may be contaminated with a wide range of carcinogens, pesticides, dioxin, antibiotic residues, synthetic hormones, etc.*

Chocolate wafer cookies: *enriched flour, sugar, vegetable shortening (partially hydrogenated soybean oil and/or cottonseed oil), cocoa (processed with alkali), high fructose corn syrup, coconut preserved with sulfur dioxide, chocolate, whey, baking soda, salt, eggs, soy lecithin, dextrose, artificial flavor.*

That's over 50 different ingredients in 1 meal! It's a chemical nightmare for your digestive system, not to mention the toxicity of some of these substances.

Start reading food labels and you will quickly notice that most meals are made up of way too many ingredients. Because different foods require different digestive mediums, having numerous ingredients at the same meal increases the probability of impaired digestion.

A good way to prevent any poor combinations is to eat fewer types of food per meal. For example, if you eat fish, well don't have the rice or the potatoes...don't have dessert and don't drink anything...just eat fish! If it is salty and makes you thirsty, have tomatoes, lettuce and/or cucumber; this way, you will not be tempted to drink water, digestion will occur unimpaired and it'll even add a little variety to your meal.

GUIDELINE NO.10: Avoid Drinking with Your Meals

We humans are designed to eat high-water content foods, like fresh fruits, vegetables and sprouts. Any other foods are low-water content, and eating these makes us thirsty. *Drinking with your meals dilutes digestive juices, consequently impairing digestion and whisking undigested food particles prematurely from the stomach to the small intestine.* Even just one cup of coffee, a glass of water or a glass of wine taken regularly with meals, for example, is enough to contribute to weight gain over time. If you increase the overall proportions of high-water content foods in your dietary, you will be generally less thirsty. Eating high-water content non-starchy vegetables (e.g., celery, cucumber, bell pepper and lettuce) along with low-water content foods (e.g., meat, fish, pasta and bread) helps quench thirst without hindering digestion.

It is also important to know that beverages, taken with or without food, are either "healthy" or "weight-promoting". It's OK to drink healthy ones without food, but you need to also reduce your overall intake of weight-promoting ones.

HEALTHY BEVERAGES	WEIGHT-PROMOTING BEVERAGES
Coconut juice	Alcohol
Extracted juices (e.g., carrot juice)	Carbonated drinks (e.g., soft drinks)
Freshly blended (e.g., banana & mango)	Coffee
Freshly squeezed (e.g., orange)	Milk
Maple water	Tea & herbal teas
Water	
	Beverages with additives (sugars, flavors, colors, electrolytes, etc.)
	Processed beverages (pasteurized, from concentrate, boiled, steamed, etc.)
	All other beverages that are not listed

GUIDELINE NO.11: Reduce Your Intake of Refined Sugars and Flours

The refining process of food items is the act of extracting one or a few food elements from their original place of creation in order to make a concentrated batch of the said elements. For example, white refined sugar comes from sugar beets or sugar cane, whereas the more popular refined flours come from cereals. In both cases, the final products have high-sugar content. The problem with eating refined sugars and refined flours is that it causes carbohydrate excesses, *which the body then turns into fat*. Sugar is vital but, in excess, is fattening. Examples of popular refined foods are:

- white and brown sugar
- most flours
- vegetable oils
- white rice
- concentrated fruit juices
- food made with any of the above-listed items (i.e., breads, pastries, pasta, cookies, doughnuts, cakes, muffins, French fries, chips, pizza, salad dressings, sauce mix, crackers, corn syrup, molasses, candy bars and most chocolates)

"Reducing"

As you will notice, some guidelines in Step 3 specify reducing something in your dietary. It is important that you don't get all panicky because you think you just read the word eliminate. Granted, *elimination* is a form of *reduction*, but it's not the only one. There's a whole spectrum of actions that correspond to the word *reduction*. So don't be scared that you have to *completely eliminate* certain foods from your dietary...the idea is to find the right progression that gives the wanted results...not too much to discourage, but enough to produce weight loss.

We suggest you keep a journal of weekly habits; this way, it'll be easy to see if you have been reducing the intake of weight-promoting foods or not. Keeping a journal doesn't have to be complicated: you simply need, for example, to indicate whether or not refined sugar/ flour was present at a given meal, and then calculate the weekly total in order to *reduce* the following week. You may also do the same to keep track of the following Guidelines that include reducing other types of foods. Refer to the *Recommended Eating Guidelines Checklist* at the end of this chapter; use one everyday to create your journal.

GUIDELINE NO.12: Reduce Your Intake of "Non-Foods"

Our bodies are designed to digest and assimilate *clean* ("clean" as in free of pesticides, hormones, antibiotics, preservatives, colorants, flavor enhancers, etc.), *fresh*, *raw*, *non-processed* and *organic* foods. Most items at your local food store are highly processed and, because processing tends to destroy nutrients, do not possess these characteristics. Such items (breakfast cereals, breads, cookies, pasta, canned foods, frozen dinners, chips, juice, candy, sauces, condiments, cakes, ice cream, etc.) are what we call "non-foods," and ingesting them contributes greatly to weight gain.

The "food" industry goes to great lengths to produce packaging that makes such "non-food" items appealing as you walk through the grocery aisles, but please, don't fall prey to this marketing. Use your common sense and start reducing your intake of non-foods.

GUIDELINE NO.13: Reduce Your Intake of Animal Products

By design, animals produce more substances (e.g., cholesterol and saturated fats) deemed toxic by our digestive system than living organisms from the plant world. Also, because animals are at the end of the food chain, the probabilities of toxins concentrating in their tissues are greater than in plants. In the food chain, for example, phytoplankton (aquatic plants) will be eaten by shrimp, which will be eaten by bleak (fish), which will be eaten by perch (a bigger fish), which will be eaten by northern pike (even bigger fish), which will finally be eaten by humans. Even in an ideal world, free of environmental pollutants, the amount of toxins concentrated from one organism to the next would result in a toxin level not recommended for our weight loss goal of reducing toxin intake...but we do not live in such a clean world, so we end up eating animals full of both naturally produced toxins and environmental pollutants.

In the food industry, the problem gets compounded as mass quantities of antibiotics, growth hormones, colorants, preservative agents and a host of other chemicals are added, making toxin levels increasingly more alarming. Cows, for example, are fed an array of substances that, over time, concentrate in their tissues; we then eat their flesh or consume their products (milk, cheese, clabber, yogurt, cream, butter, ice cream, etc.). Cows are also fed grass sprayed with pesticides, and these too amass in their flesh tissues; sometimes, cows are even fed crushed and powdered parts of other animals, giving way to diseases such as mad cow disease.

In order to apply this guideline, here is a suggestion: firstly assess your current intake of animal products (e.g., the number of meals per week that have such products in them) and then, from week to week, decrease this amount as much as possible; by doing this, you will be reducing your toxin intake and thus promoting weight loss.

Of course, as you diminish your intake of animal products, you may have the following preoccupation...

"What About My Protein?"

Contrary to what you've been told, we *do not* need protein in our dietary. I know, I know, this may come as a big surprise and shock you into disbelief, but ask any physician and they will agree with the following: we need proteins to function as human beings, and our cells make them, so we do not need to ingest any; what we do need, so that our cells can manufacture proteins, are amino acids, as found in most foods from the plant world (not the amino acids used as body building supplements. . . that's another story).

Eating animal products as a source of amino acids is not ideal because:

Of the extra digestive steps and additional energy required to break down proteins into their constituents (amino acids); in food from the plant world, amino acids are readily available.

Of their high levels of toxin, which are much higher than those in food from the plant world.

Most animal products require cooking; this process coagulates and clumps proteins together, making their digestion very difficult.

Condiments, sauces and a host of other substances are needed to make animal products appealing, thus increasing the probabilities of chemical incompatibilities and thwarted digestion.

Therefore, as you reduce your intake of animal products in order to lose weight (and become healthier), don't worry about not getting your protein. Follow the Recommended Eating Guidelines and you'll have more than enough protein in your system.

GUIDELINE NO.14: Reduce Your Intake of Irritants

Foods like onions, leeks, garlic, spices, pepper, salt, etc., contain substances that irritate the mucosa (inner lining) of the digestive tract, causing impaired digestion and water retention. Ideally, you would want to eliminate these food items completely from your dietary, but because many such irritants are found in a great deal of recipes, it may be difficult to eliminate them altogether; consequently, aim to *decrease* their consumption as much as possible.

Here are a few examples:

IRRITANTS

Chives	Radish
Garlic	Salt
Leek	Scallion
Parsley	Spices
Onion	Watercress
Pepper	

GUIDELINE NO.15: Reduce Your Intake of Cooked Foods

Cooking often destroys nutrients or transforms certain benign elements into toxic ones; this contributes to the body's toxic load. If you reduce your intake of cooked foods, look to increase your intake of raw wholesome living foods, like non-processed fresh fruits, vegetables, sprouts, nuts and seeds. Because we are used to cooked foods being high in gustatory stimulation, it is important to find the tastiest of raw foods, or else you will find your new dietary quite bland, and integrating this guideline will fail.

When looking for tasty produce, do not limit yourself only to bulk fruits and vegetables from bigger supermarkets, as these tend to be less flavorful; visit also smaller local produce shops or health food stores with lots of organic varieties.

We've added a recipe section to this book to give you a few helpful suggestions as you discover this new healthy way of eating. Eating to promote weight loss and to simplify weight control can be just as tasty as anything you have ever had!

GUIDELINE NO.16: Do Not Overeat

Easy to say but not always easy to do, right? Here, then, are a few tips to make it easier:

- **Know That You May Be Eating Just to Compensate for a Lack of Healthy Stimulation.**

Sitting in traffic, working at a desk, answering a phone 40 hours a week, trying to meet project deadlines, cramming for exams, being stressed at work, mowing the lawn...such less-than-stimulating activities often lead to *"I need to spoil myself a little now"*, and so we reach for food. Most of the time, we're not even aware that we eat to make up for life's dull moments, but food is simple and easily accessible, and this leads to overeating.

In order to avoid overeating, catch yourself when you're about to eat for the *sole purpose* of reward, and quickly look for fulfillment in some other way. Search for new options to balance out unhealthy stimulation with healthy stimulation, like going for a walk, sex, exercise, a good book, a massage, a movie or a shopping spree. Find whatever works for you.

- **Stop Eating When 80% Full.**

When you have a meal, it takes about 20 minutes for the stretch receptors in your stomach to register the full weight of what you have just eaten. These receptors then tell your brain, but by this time, you have already overeaten. Ever get that feeling that you feel fuller after a meal than during? That's why. A good habit to develop, therefore, is to eat to approximately 80% capacity, wait a good 20 minutes, and then, *if you are still hungry*, eat some more. In addition, don't stuff yourself simply because there's some left in your plate...starting something doesn't justify finishing it.

- **Increase Your Proportion of Healthy Foods.**

Although the answer to the question *"How do we become hungry?"* is still not well understood by science, one of the possible factors is the monitoring of blood nutrients by the brain. If these nutrients decrease, your brain produces a hunger sensation; if you've just finished a meal and there is no increase in nutrients, your brain also produces a hunger sensation. Here lies the problem with most of our eating habits: we eat foods void of nutrients (e.g., processed foods, junk food and non-foods), or have ill-combined meals (as explained earlier, causing nutrient loss), and so the quantity of nutrients in the blood *does not increase*.

This scares the body, because eating is the process by which the levels of nutrients are *supposed* to increase. As a result, this scenario produces hunger again, and again, until the levels of nutrients increase. Overeating usually occurs at this point. Low-nutrient foods or ill-combined meals provide the body with very little usable nutrients and produce a high quantity of waste. On the other hand, fresh raw organic foods provide our system with a greater quantity of usable substances (over time, and not simply after a few servings, of course...). As you integrate the Recommended Eating Guidelines, you will notice that you eat less; this is due to the higher quality of foods and the proper handling and serving of meals.

- **Increase Overall Healthy Activities.**

  Making your eating habits healthier ones will get you to lose weight, but don't stop there. If you also begin to transform other areas of your life, like exercise, rest, stress management, fun, etc., your body will get even cleaner, fitter and stronger. As this occurs, weight-promoting foods and compulsive eating will be less tempting

- **Know That Excess Protein Will Turn into Fat.**

  We all know that consuming excess fat or sugar causes weight gain, but did you also know that the body turns excess protein into fat? People still believe that ingesting large quantities of protein will cause muscle growth, but the body actually turns excess protein into fat. Because protein is very common in today's foods, one has to be careful not to create any excesses. To get an idea of your consumption, keep a journal for 2 weeks detailing your protein intake, and then make the appropriate changes. Again, use the Checklist at the end of the chapter to create this journal.

- **Take a Good Look at the Amount of Food in Your Plate Before Ingesting It.**

  Get into the habit of taking a good look at the quantity of food that you're about to ingest at a given meal (include all: starters, appetizers, beverages, dessert, etc.) and ask yourself: *"Do I really need to put that much food into my stomach?"* Ask this question before every meal until it becomes second nature. Most of us eat too much anyway but, as mentioned previously, we only find out approximately 20 minutes later. I suggest that you eat smaller meals and, if you feel you must, eat more often; for example, divide the quantity of 3 daily meals into 6 daily meals.

GUIDELINE NO.17: Do Not Eat When Tired

The digestion and assimilation of most foods require energy. You therefore do not want to add a chore that requires energy to an already tired body. One of the numerous ongoing tasks of the body is waste management, and if energy must be diverted from this task to attend to

71

newly ingested food, wastes may not be dealt with properly and weight gain will ensue. As a rule of thumb, if you feel like taking a nap, then you're too tired to eat... go for the nap instead.

GUIDELINE NO.18: Do Not Go to Sleep with Food in Your Stomach

There is a common notion that eating before going to sleep will cause weight gain. This is a notion of high controversy. Numerous sources conclude against, some for; my experience with weight loss programs since 1996 concludes for.

My theory: waste elimination is one of the many physiological processes that occur during sleep; this elimination helps to reduce weight and keep the weight off, so if anything hinders sleep, it also hinders elimination, and then toxins accumulate inside the body and weight gain occurs.

"Does digestion hinder sleep?" Well, digestion puts your body in a state of high-energy expenditure when, as you are trying to fall asleep, it should actually be in a relaxed and calm state; this is why eating before going to bed impairs sleep and consequently promotes weight gain. Use the information from this section to determine your gastric evacuation times and proper food combinations in order to avoid having food in your stomach at bedtime.

Setting Up the Context for Your New Way of Eating

"I shall now attempt to eat a diet lunch consisting of one leaf of lettuce lightly seasoned with...one quart of mayonnaise!"
— **Garfield the cat**

Relearning how to eat is self-education; in other words, local schools are not going to teach you the contents of this chapter. How you re-train yourself to eat will be *very* different than how the world in which you live eats, so we recommend that you set up your life and schedule in a way to increase the probabilities of success. Here are a few things you can do:

- **Clean Out Your Food Stocks (Refrigerator, Kitchen Cupboards/Pantry, etc.).**

  Keep what's healthy and throw out what's unhealthy. Don't save that ketchup bottle, bag of chips or those ill-combined frozen dinners for a "cheat" occasion; not having them around will make it less tempting.

- **In the Beginning, Stay Away from Restaurants and Social Events (Which Include Food and/or Beverages) As Much As Possible.**

  I'm not saying to never go to a restaurant or have a social drink *ever again*, but try to reduce *as much as possible* initially. Once you master this book's principles and guidelines, then it'll be safer for you to venture out.

- **Prepare Your Family and Friends.**

  Get them to promise they will support you before you start your program or you'll see just how much encouragement "loved ones" give naturally. In addition, get yourself a weight loss buddy as a good source of motivation. See if there is anyone in your entourage who would like to lose weight, and do the program together; it's always easier if you have someone supporting you, and it keeps you walking a straight line knowing that someone else will be checking in on you. In fact, making a promise to someone else is often more powerful than only to ourselves.

- **Quickly Integrate New Exercise and Sleeping Habits to Complement and Support Your New Way of Eating.**

  Balance out the other parts of your schedule as rapidly as possible so you are not tempted to turn to food as a solution to unfulfilled stimulation. Make it a good strong start.

- **"Cheat" As Little As Possible.**

  Goes without say, right? If you do deviate, however, then *transition back* to the Recommended Eating Guidelines as hard and as quickly as possible. When you "deviate" or "cheat" (as in an "ill-combined meal"), *transitioning back* means to eat nothing for as many hours as possible in order to give your stomach a chance to empty itself (i.e., to evacuate the spoiling food) and to thus create a context for efficient digestion. "As many hours as possible" does not mean days on end, of course, but usually in the vicinity of 6 to 8 hours (this does not include sleeping or exercise time). Here's a little more on the subject...

Transitioning Back After Having "Cheated"

It is important to allow for a transition period after having "cheated" in order to give your body a chance not to fall behind in its waste management tasks, and to be able to eliminate the toxic load caused by an ill-combined meal. You would *ideally* want to wait 6 to 8 hours—"wait" in this context meaning "not eat anything." *Always calculate this waiting period from the time you finished eating, and not from the time you started your meal.*

If you find the waiting period too long, and you *absolutely positively cannot wait any longer* and must eat, then have a salad made up of neutral ("neutral" as in no sugar and no acid) high-water content vegetables such as lettuce, celery and cucumber. Sounds boring? Well, maybe, but it's one way to deal with a long wait; if you were to eat anything else, it would only go to waste on top of the already spoiling food.

Another way to deal with the wait is to drink water; although not ideal because it will dilute digestive juices and delay digestion, water is neutral and, if drinking some prevents you from eating more food, then it's a step in the right direction.

Yet another way of dealing with a long transition period is to drink caffeinated beverages...that's right, caffeinated beverages (coffee, tea, Red Bull, Coke, Pepsi, etc.), because caffeine and caffeine-like stimulants (theine, guaranine, etc.) induce gastric evacuation. Now, don't see this as a cure-all for "cheating"; in other words, it's not because you know caffeine stimulates gastric evacuation that you should permit yourself to "cheat" more often... this would be like intentionally hitting your head against a wall knowing you can take a Tylenol shortly after...kinda defeats the purpose of wanting to be healthy, doesn't it?

During the wait, it is better to be awake and slightly active, as opposed to lying in bed asleep; "awake" means digestion will continue, and "active" (as in walking, moving around, etc., but not exercising because this suspends digestive processes) helps with the mechanical aspect of digestion. In time, as you become healthier, your body will be able to deal with "cheat" occasions more efficiently, making for shorter transition periods.

• Approximately 3-4 hours after the ill-combined meal, you'll have "the munchies" (i.e., a light feeling of wanting to nibble on something). At this point, do not eat! Resist temptation.

• 3-4 hours after that (so 6-8 hours after the meal), you will experience movement in your stomach and a feeling of thirst mixed with salivation. This usually lasts 10-15 minutes. I always feel like my digestive tract is pushing the remainder of the meal to the intestines where it will be processed for elimination. At this point, your stomach is ready for new food.

- **Budget Permitting, Don't Hesitate to Invest in Healthy Foods.**

  Organic items may have a higher price tag than other foods, but if they help with weight loss, aren't they suddenly worth it? As the cashier tallies up my grocery bill, I often remind myself: *"It's OK, it's a health investment...it's OK, it's a health investment..."*

- **Look to Create Varied Meals.**

  Eating the same one or two things at first will be tempting because of its simplicity, but quickly look for variety, as this will increase your chances of success.

- **Always Have Healthy Food Handy.**

  Or else you'll want to rapidly satisfy an urge and end up creating a full meal from the office vending machine...

- **Put Failsafe Mechanisms into Place to Be Ready When Temptation Strikes.**

  In moments of strong temptation, I usually stop, take a few deep breaths, and see if I can't persuade myself not to give in: *"If I eat the fried chicken now, how long will this pleasure last? Is 10-15 minutes of gustatory pleasure worth 6-8 hours of digestion? Is eating before going to bed worth impairing a good night's sleep? Is the amount of money I'm going to spend on alcohol worth the impact it'll have on my budget and on my health?"* Find out what *your* failsafe mechanisms are and use them readily.

A Final Note to Step 3

"The big secret in life is that there is no big secret. Whatever your goal, you can get there if you're willing to work."
— **Oprah Winfrey**
first African American woman to become a billionaire

Now that you have read Step 3, you may be thinking...

"It's too complicated, so I'll find another way..."

"Man, it's way too restrictive...I wouldn't be able to eat anything anymore!"

"That's crazy; no one can eat this way!"

"What am I supposed to eat?"

And these are all perfectly understandable and valid reactions.

Consider, however, that reactions and points of view are always in reference to something specific; your point of view on the information contained in this chapter is in reference to what you have been conditioned to believe constitutes "healthy eating," and this is why our Recommended Eating Guidelines may seem extreme, restrictive and not worth the effort. Food notions are strong and, as far as you're concerned, they are THE TRUTH. It makes sense. Think about it for just a minute: what you know about food and healthy eating has been part of your life both theoretically and experientially for as long as you've been alive...what your parents, teachers and doctors have taught you...what you've read and learned from books and magazines...what you've experienced through diets and fitness programs...and here we are, Helene and I, complete strangers, asking you to now consider a different reality. Our point of view is based on years of successfully designing weight loss programs and managing our own weight to perfection, so, as far as we're concerned, the information from Step 3 is far from being extreme. Unconventional and challenging maybe, but not extreme, and most definitely worth the effort.

To conclude, know this: even after years of integrating and perfecting healthy eating habits, Helene and I's dietary still does not correspond 100% to what you have read in this chapter: we eat very healthy, and then we cheat some...and then we eat very healthy again, and then we allow ourselves to cheat some more...etc. We know that weight loss and weight management are a function of what one does as a rule, and not as the exception. I thus suggest you see the Recommended Eating Guidelines as "something to aim for", and not as "a discipline hammer with which to hit yourself every time you're not respecting these Guidelines"; the trick is to eat in a way that gives desired results. If you REALLY want to create weight loss in a *safe*, *balanced*, *healthy* and *sustainable* way, you have to start to apply the Recommended Eating Guidelines. Do it progressively and find the pace that works for you. I'm 20 years into it and still find myself having to resist society's weight-promoting temptations...every day! When faced with such temptations and as a rule, however, my choice to maintain a healthy weight wins over giving in to weight-promoting foods.

The choice is now yours...

Recommended Eating Guidelines

1.   Respect gastric evacuation times.

2.   Do not eat proteins and fats/oils at same meal.

3.   Do not eat proteins and starchy foods at same meal.

4.   Do not eat proteins and sweet foods at same meal.

5.   Do not eat starchy foods and acid foods at same meal.

6.   Do not eat fruits with any other type of food.

7.   Eat melons only with other melons, nothing else.

8.   Do not eat sweet fruits with acid fruits.

9.   Simplify your meals.

10. Avoid drinking with your meals.

11. Reduce your intake of refined foods.

12. Reduce your intake of "non-foods."

13. Reduce your intake of animal products.

14. Reduce your intake of irritants.

15. Reduce your intake of cooked foods.

16. Do not overeat.

17. Do not eat when tired.

18. Do not go to sleep with food in your stomach.

Date: _____

Simply insert a 🙂 , 🙁 or "N/A" (for "not applicable") in the appropriate cells.

	Breakfast	Snack	Lunch	Snack	Dinner	Snack
Stomach ready for this meal?						
Protein & fat/oil at same meal?						
Protein & starchy food at same meal?						
Protein & sweet food at same meal?						
Starchy food & acid food at same meal?						
Fruit with any other type of food?						
Melon & non-melon at same meal?						
Sweet fruit & acid fruit at same meal?						
Meal simplified?						
Any beverage(s) with this meal?						

Any refined foods at this meal?						
Any "non-foods" at this meal?						
Any animal products at this meal?						
Any irritants at this meal?						
Any cooked foods at this meal?						
Did I overeat? (Be honest)						
Was I tired when I ate this meal?						
Did I have food in my stomach as I went to sleep?						

Food Combining Chart

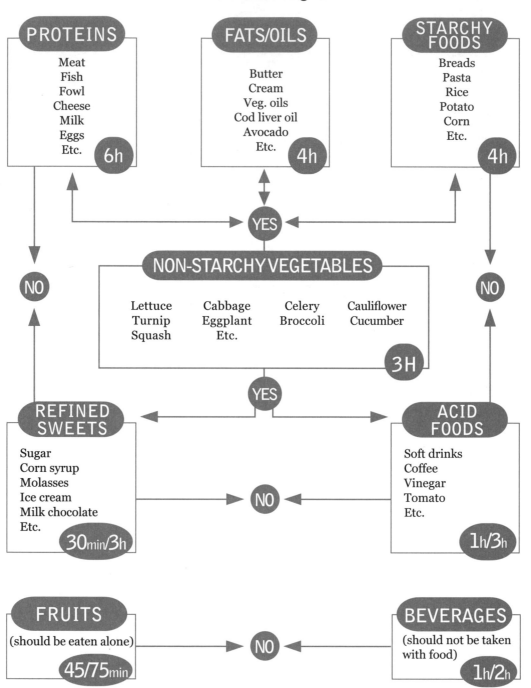

PROTEINS
Meat
Fish
Fowl
Cheese
Milk
Eggs
Etc.
6h

FATS/OILS
Butter
Cream
Veg. oils
Cod liver oil
Avocado
Etc.
4h

STARCHY FOODS
Breads
Pasta
Rice
Potato
Corn
Etc.
4h

YES

NON-STARCHY VEGETABLES
Lettuce   Cabbage   Celery   Cauliflower
Turnip   Eggplant   Broccoli Cucumber
Squash   Etc.
3H

NO

NO

YES

REFINED SWEETS
Sugar
Corn syrup
Molasses
Ice cream
Milk chocolate
Etc.
30min/3h

NO

ACID FOODS
Soft drinks
Coffee
Vinegar
Tomato
Etc.
1h/3h

FRUITS
(should be eaten alone)
45/75min

NO

BEVERAGES
(should not be taken with food)
1h/2h

Fruit Combining Chart

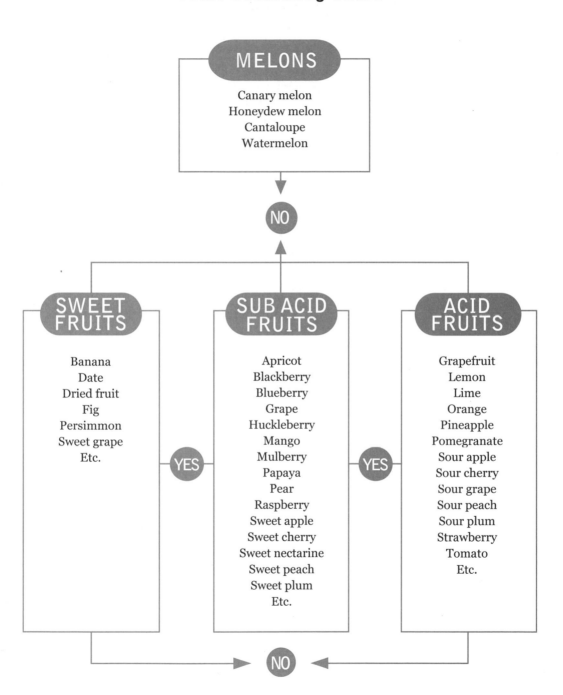

MELONS

Canary melon
Honeydew melon
Cantaloupe
Watermelon

NO

SWEET FRUITS

Banana
Date
Dried fruit
Fig
Persimmon
Sweet grape
Etc.

YES

SUB ACID FRUITS

Apricot
Blackberry
Blueberry
Grape
Huckleberry
Mango
Mulberry
Papaya
Pear
Raspberry
Sweet apple
Sweet cherry
Sweet nectarine
Sweet peach
Sweet plum
Etc.

YES

ACID FRUITS

Grapefruit
Lemon
Lime
Orange
Pineapple
Pomegranate
Sour apple
Sour cherry
Sour grape
Sour peach
Sour plum
Strawberry
Tomato
Etc.

NO

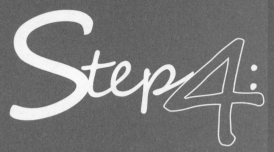

Step 4: Exercising So That it Makes a Difference

"Motivation is a fire from within. If someone else tries to light that fire under you, chances are it will burn very briefly."
— **DR. Stephen R. Covey**
best-selling author of *The Seven Habits of Highly Effective People*

"It's only work if somebody makes you do it."
— **Calvin**
of *Calvin & Hobbes Comic Books*

Because exercise and weight loss have such a well-established relationship in today's society, it would seem a little superfluous to devote an entire chapter to it. Just like popular erroneous notions on what constitutes "healthy eating," however, we have found that many individuals are *convinced* they are exercising both efficiently and sufficiently, but that they also end up being confused in the face of no weight loss results: *"I exercise a lot, and I'm sure I do it right, but it never seems to make a big difference...I don't understand!?...I'm putting a lot of effort into it, so why am I not losing weight!?"*

Let's begin by looking at your relationship to exercise. You may already be a very active person, in which case this section may act as good review material and as acknowledgment to the efforts you are and have been putting toward physical activity...as you read, you'll be able to say, *"Hey, I already do this, I'm pretty good!"* You may, on the other hand, be more of a sedentary nature, and so the information that follows will be very useful. You may also *think* that you are *sufficiently* active to cause weight loss, but you'll discover as you read on that your activity level may need a little bit of a boost. Either way, enjoy.

In a nutshell, exercise equals waste elimination, and that's the weight-loss value we are seeking through physical activity.

In order to exercise so that it makes a difference, we suggest you focus on the following 4 aspects:

1. Type
2. Frequency
3. Intensity
4. Motivation

Type

"Happiness is not achieved by the conscious pursuit of happiness; it is generally the by-product of other activities."
— **Aldous Huxley**
Writer

The type of exercise needed for weight loss often goes beyond household chores, errands or physical jobs. You may break a sweat by gardening, raking leaves or cleaning the tub, but that's not enough. You may perform hard work or heavy labor at your job, but that's usually not sufficient either. Of course, there's nothing wrong with using chores, errands and work to burn off a few calories, but if the goal is weight loss, then you need to partake in a vigorous and formal exercise program.

If you have never partaken regularly in a formal exercise program, please keep in mind that a sudden change in lifestyle may be difficult. It doesn't have to be difficult, but it may. Because losing weight is a goal YOU have chosen freely, however, incorporating a new exercise program as part of your weekly routine does not have to appear as something arduously imposed. In other words, it can be fun!

Motivation is the most important element of success. We recommend you pick a type of physical activity that seems appealing. Do not partake in a specific type of physical activity just because it's in vogue. You have to find your own motivation, or else it will not stick.

Progression is also important, so do not attempt to run a marathon within the first week. It took years for you to put on extra weight, so give yourself at least a few weeks to take it off. Progression is the surest way for you to avoid injuries and to remain motivated. For example, if you joined an organized sport and felt that the intensity was too much for your present fitness level, then it would be wiser to choose something else. You could always come back to this particular sport once you had *progressed* to its level.

Moreover, *don't be shy to get experienced help*, in order not to hurt yourself and to get the most out of it. Find an expert for your type of exercise, an expert being someone with more experience than you (professional trainer, a friend, etc.). Get guidelines, and make sure it respects the *frequency* and *intensity* as described further in this chapter.

A type of exercise we highly recommend for beginners is walking. Yes, that's right, walking. Walking is safe for people of all ages and in all states of health. It requires no specific equipment (other than a good pair of shoes) or specific venue, and it produces a host of health benefits. The other added feature is that walking can be easily incorporated into anyone's schedule: walk to work, walk to the store, walk to a friend's home, etc. For walking to be effective, however, it must also respect our recommended *intensity* and *frequency* guidelines. In order to increase the intensity, for example, walk up hill or walk with a small weight in your hands and/or around your ankles.

In regards to your overall weekly exercise program, increase the intensity and incorporate other types of activities so as to solicit all 3 of the following components:

- Lung and heart capacity (e.g., jogging and swimming)
- Muscular development (e.g., weights, push-ups and sit-ups)
- Flexibility (e.g., yoga and stretching)

Aim to cover these components with all activities combined, and not necessarily through one given activity. Some activities may solicit more than one component, of course; swimming, for example, works lungs, heart (cardiovascular) *and* muscular development. Some types of yoga, on the other hand, focus on flexibility *and* muscular development. It is not ideal to develop only one component while neglecting others (as is often the case with weight lifters, for example, where muscular development is emphasized, but cardio and flexibility are neglected). Like always, strive for balance.

Frequency

"You may have to fight a battle more than once to win it."
— **Margaret Thatcher**
first and only woman to date to hold both posts of Prime
Minister of the U.K. and Leader of the British Conservative Party

Question: *How often should I exercise during my weight loss program?*
Answer: *Every day. That's correct. EVERY DAY.*

OK, OK, I can just hear the *"But that's crazy, I don't have time!"* Listen, do you want to lose weight or not?

If exercise has not been a regular part of your lifestyle, then there is a psychological barrier that you must overcome. You'll need to jump into this weight loss program with a "no kidding" attitude or else your conditioned sedentary side will dominate. The quicker you get results, the more motivated you will be to continue exercising. Another advantage to daily exercise is the proximity of the sessions, for having those far apart gives your psyche more time to find excuses not to make it to the next one. You do not want this. You want results. You want to feel proud and look like a million bucks.

I recommend that, as you begin the program, you exercise every day for a period of 1 hour, divided in the following manner:

- 10-minute warm-up period
- 40 minutes of vigorous activity
- 10-minute cool-down period.

I also recommend you exercise in the morning because:

A - you have more energy and
B - once it's done, it's done.

Nothing can suddenly appear in your schedule that would make you miss your session; you can't ignore it or postpone it, or surprisingly "run out of time" later in the day.

In order to increase your chances of being assiduous, schedule sessions in advance and get an exercise buddy. Imagine the not-too-distant future, looking back in the pages of your organizer and being proud of having had exercise as a daily activity, and thus having lost a good deal of weight...sounds encouraging, doesn't it? Make a promise to yourself now, and honor it; keeping your word builds self-confidence and establishes good credibility with yourself for any future endeavors. Think about it: people that make good on their promises inspire trust. The same is true for us with ourselves: honoring our word builds self-confidence, even if it's toward what may seem trivial at times, like regular exercise, fixing things around the house, cleaning up and tidying the car and work station, etc. See how many things are not yet done (and, for some reason, keep not getting done...) on your to-do list, and get to them.

One of the goals of this daily routine is to work up metabolism so that you can eventually afford to skip a few planned weekly exercise sessions, without losing your shape. Train your body to operate at such a high level of health that it will fair very well on only *occasional* sessions. Take Olympic athletes, for example: their bodies are such clean, well-run and fine-tuned machines that occasionally skipping a work out, or even indulging in the odd unhealthy activity (e.g., eating junk food), will not affect their state of health. I'm not saying you have to be an Olympic athlete to attain a high level of health, but start training and conditioning your body so that it can also afford to slack off once in a while and still maintain a perfectly healthy weight...it's an awesome feeling, trust me.

Intensity

"Some people want it to happen, some wish it would happen, others make it happen."

— **Michael Jordan**

Be vigorous enough to produce the desired outcome (in this case losing weight), but not too vigorous so as to cause injury. In other words, push yourself, but don't hurt yourself. Midway into the session, you should feel that:

- Your respiratory rate has gone up significantly.
- Your heart rate has also gone up significantly.
- You have produced a good sweat.

Granted, words like "significantly" and "good" have relative meanings, so here are a few guidelines:

- **Consider Hiring a Professional Trainer.**

  A good way to get an initial fitness appraisal, and to make sure you are doing it safely and effectively, is to get professional help. A trainer is able to assess your starting point, with tools like the Physical Activity Readiness Questionnaire or Physical Activity Readiness Medical Examination, or tests like VO2 Max, which measures your aerobic capacity. A host of other evaluations are available to properly determine your starting point and keep track of your progress.

- **Be Panting and Somewhat "Out-of-Breath" During and Immediately After Your Session.**

  I've known individuals who were certain that walking a few miles every day was enough to get their system to eliminate extra weight. They walked on flat ground, however, and their pace was so slow and effortless that not a drop of sweat and no visible signs of exhaustion were present...as if they had just come out of the library! If you're going to invest time and energy in physical activity so as to cause weight loss, you'll have to push yourself a little more than that. A good measure to ensure this is to exercise between 60% and 85% of your Maximum Heart Rate (MHR).

"What Is My Maximum Heart Rate?"

Well, it's very simple: to figure out your MHR, subtract your age from 220. For example, if you are 40, your MHR is 180 (220 minus 40 years old).

In order to work up your intensity progressively, begin by exercising at 60% of your MHR. If your MHR is 180, then you need to exercise at 108 beats per minute (180 MHR x 60%). In order to evaluate your effort, measure your beats per minute during your workout, called your Active Heart Rate.

Measuring Your Active Heart Rate

To measure this in beats per minute (BPM), stop halfway into your exercise session and find your pulse (either at the wrist or on the side of your throat). Do not use your thumb because it has a pulse of its own; use any other finger. With a watch or a clock handy, count beats for 10 seconds, multiply this by 6, and this gives your heart rate in beats per minute.

With each exercise session, increase your MHR percentage, moving from 60% up toward 85%. If your health is fragile, or if you have any concerns, please consult with your physician before undertaking any type of physical activity.

A quick and easy reference to know if you're pushing yourself hard enough is that, *during* your session, you should find it difficult to hold a conversation.

- **Don't Aim to Lose Weight By Sweating in a Sauna.**

  Here's the thing to know: sweating in a sauna is not the same as sweating through vigorous exercise. If you're sitting and it's hot (like in a sauna, hot tub or outside on a hot summer day), mostly water is coming out and practically no toxins. Thus, sitting in a sauna (or doing yoga in a sauna) will get you to lose weight, but mostly by water loss. If you exercise with intensity, on the other hand, water and *a host of toxins* are eliminated from your body. For weight loss purposes, you want the latter.

- **You Should Feel Muscle Soreness the Next Day.**

  This is called Delayed Onset Muscle Soreness (D.O.M.S.), and it is perfectly normal to experience after having had a good hard workout. In time, your body will get fitter and D.O.M.S. will not appear as readily or as often.

  There is a popular saying *"No pain, no gain."* Although some discomfort in the form of muscular soreness is nothing to fear and can even be a way to measure one's work effort, I do not recommend that you try to produce this at all cost. It is very possible to exercise vigorously without being sore the next day. As mentioned previously, rule of thumb is: push yourself but don't hurt yourself.

- **Keep in Mind That Shorter Periods of More Intense Activity Are Better than Longer Periods of Milder Activity.**

  You'll benefit more, for example, by running hard for 40 minutes than moderately for 60 minutes.

Motivation

"Pain is temporary. Quitting lasts forever."
— **Lance Armstrong**
won a record-breaking seven consecutive Tour de France after
recovering from battling cancer

If you want to look forward to your next exercise session, and if you want the experience of doing physical activity to be stimulating and fun, it is very important to find sources of motivation. These are as varied as there are different individuals. What motivates you may not motivate the next person, and vice versa. It is important to identify what fuels *your* enthusiasm for physical activity. Use the following criteria when considering integrating exercise as a regular lifestyle component:

- **Type**: Is this type of exercise well suited for my needs? For my health? Am I having fun?
- **Cost**: Can I afford it? Are costs going to add stress to my life?
- **Accessibility**: Is it easy for me to get to or do I have to drive far?
- **Time requirements**: Can I fit it easily into my schedule?

If you find a type of activity you really enjoy, chances are that cost, accessibility and time requirements will fall into place. Motivation will be present and you will make it happen. As previously mentioned, do not choose a type of exercise because it is trendy; do not let that be the determining factor.

Aside from type of exercise, type of venue can also be influential. For example, I much prefer jogging in forest trails than on a gym treadmill. I may have to drive some distance to get to the forest, but for me, it's worth it. That is my personal preference; identify yours.

If you look long and hard and still cannot find anything, then simply choose one. Start by choosing the best of the "worst," or the one with the most potential of becoming fun, and funnel your search results by trial and error. Weight loss results will prove to be inspirational enough to develop the required motivation.

Finding motivation reminds me of a young bird in a nest, just waiting for its mother to push it out so it can learn to fly. Human adults are very much like the little bird, often waiting for someone to push them into their own lives. The difference with human adults, however, is that there is no Mama Bird to push us; as grown-ups, we are responsible for our own initiatives. We have to find the *courage* to jump, and only then can we experience life by leaving the confines of our nest and soaring in the blue skies.

Courage

Courage is not "making the fear go away so we can then proceed." Courage is firstly acknowledging fear, and then going through with what we set out to do. For example, if someone is afraid of public speaking but needs to get up in front of an audience and speak, well, that person will simply acknowledge the presence of fear, and get up there and speak. In order not to be stopped, one has to make the motivation behind both commitments and goals bigger than the fear.

If you are keen to begin a new exercise program but still hesitate, simply acknowledge your fears, and get your goals accomplished nonetheless. If going through life and being overweight is not your idea of fun, then get to it. You don't get a practice life... this is no rehearsal, so make it count!

Another recommendation when it comes to exercise is *to be result oriented*. Don't let petty things get in the way. I once knew someone who let pride and fear of tainting her self-image be obstacles; she wanted to take up running, but didn't want her neighbors to see her running in the streets. She eventually mustered up the courage to get some nice jogging clothes and shoes, and went out strutin' her stuff. Pride went from being an obstacle to being a main source of motivation, especially when, 2 months later, she had lost over 30 pounds!

You want to be able to always look back to the past and be proud of having had physical activity as a regular occurrence. Don't let all the good reasons, like *"I don't have enough time"*, *"I don't feel like it"* or *"I can't find a type of exercise I like"* justify being lazy. NO WAY! You're an adult...DO WHAT IT TAKES. You want to adopt a "no kidding" attitude toward this program. I'm not implying here that exercise should appear as discipline and hard work; in fact, I highly suggest that you find ways to make it just the opposite, light and playful.

In your quest to get results, consider the following: *the key to achieving your goals lies in the ability to perform the acts aligned with the results envisioned.*

Q & A

Question: *Is weight loss possible without exercise?*
Answer: *Yes.*

Question: *Is it OK if I skip the exercise part of the weight loss program and focus instead on food and the other components?*
Answer: *No.*

Achieving goals is a question of probabilities. Given that we live in a society that promotes weight gain, we have to increase our chances of succeeding at weight loss by focusing on ALL components (i.e., food, exercise, sleep and stress management). This way, weight reduction has a greater chance of occurring.

Question: *How long will it take before I tone up and stay firm?*
Answer: *It depends.*

Depending on their genetic predisposition, some people tone up quicker than others. Certain individuals find the nice muscular definition they once had in just a few weeks, while others need to build it for the first time, and this can take months. If you're looking for fast results, please do not take any body building supplements (e.g., amino acids and whey powder) or fat-burning pills, as these create imbalances and divert valuable energy needed for toxin elimination.

One thing to keep in mind is that your muscular definition will appear more rapidly as you lose weight, and this can be very encouraging. So eat right, exercise regularly, get great sleep, create a stress-free mindset, and you will get a beautiful "bod" in no time!

Step 4 — Exercising So That it Makes a Difference

95

Exercise Checklist

Dates, from _____ to _____

Simply insert "yes," "no," "N/A" (for "not applicable") or a time &
date in the appropriate cells.

	Sun	Mon	Tue	Wed	Thu	Fri	Sat
Is this activity well suited for me?							
Am I respecting progression?							
Am I motivated to do this type of exercise?							
Have I considered getting experienced help?							
Am I using the 10 min warm-up 40 min vigorous 10 min cool-down recommendation?							
Do I exercise in the morning?							
Has my respiratory rate gone up?							
Has my heart rate gone up?							
Did I manage to produce a good sweat?							
Do I feel D.O.M.S. today?							
Was my session fun?							

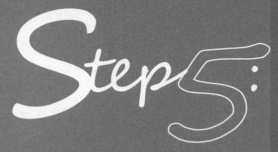

Step 5: Incorporating Sleep As a Weight Loss Element

"There are two primary choices in life; to accept conditions as they exist, or accept the responsibility for changing them."
— Dr. Denis Waitley
best-selling author, keynote speaker and productivity consultant

"Follow your own particular dreams. We are handed a life by peers, parents and society, you can do that or follow your own dreams. Life is short, be a dreamer but be a practical person."
— Hugh Hefner
founder of *Playboy*

It is common belief that little occurs during sleep, that it is a period of standstill...yet nothing could be further from the truth. Similar to what occurs during waking hours, millions of vital physiological processes also occur during sleep.

One of the main functions of sleep is the regeneration of nerve energy, very analogous to recharging a battery. In other words, we use up energy during our waking hours, so we need to regenerate it during sleep.

Another process that takes place during sleep is waste elimination. This occurs at a very high rate during periods of unconsciousness. You may notice signs of this intense elimination as you wake up in the morning with a full bladder, a pasty mouth, malodorous armpits and various other body odors. Because the name of the weight loss game is toxin elimination, it is thus essential to obtain the best possible sleep.

When aiming for best sleep, it is important to focus on *quality* and *quantity*.

Quality

"I'm much too young to feel this damn old."
– Garth Brooks

The quality of sleep for which to aim is *deep sleep*. At this level, the body is able to conduct its most efficient clean up. Poor quality sleep not only impairs waste elimination during our sleeping hours, but it also impairs it during the following waking hours. That for which to strive is better sleeping conditions, for better sleeping conditions equal better sleep.

There are both *internal* and *external* factors to the body that contribute to sleep quality:

INTERNAL FACTOR 1: Reduced Toxin Intake and Increased Toxin Elimination During Waking Hours

Because toxins deplete energy, the fewer toxins go into the body during waking hours, the less nerve regeneration is required during sleep, and thus the better the sleep. Along with waste management and nerve regeneration, there are also other vital functions that need to be accomplished during sleep - e.g., refueling the liver and cells with glycogen (a reserve sugar), destroying old cells and replacing them with new ones. A cleaner body makes it easier for *all* tasks to be performed, resulting in better recuperation and better overall health, which in turn makes waste elimination more efficient during the following days and nights.

It is recommended, of course, that all types of toxins be reduced, but *especially* those having a stimulating effect, as found in coffee (caffeine), tea (theine), sodas (caffeine, sugar, sugar supplements, etc.), energy drinks (guaranine), chocolate (caffeine, sugar), tobacco (nicotine), etc. Although stimulating initially, these toxins eventually cause nerve energy depletion. The more exhausted your body as you go to sleep, the more work it has, the fewer the chances of accomplishing all that needs to be done during that particular sleep period; in addition, a more tired body eliminates wastes less efficiently the following days and nights, and thus a vicious cycle sets in.

In addition to exhausting our system and increasing its nocturnal workload, another weight-promoting consequence of these stimulating toxins is sleep impairment, which directly affects waste elimination.

On top of reducing toxin intake, one should also look to increase toxin elimination during waking hours by way of exercise and rest (e.g., naps).

INTERNAL FACTOR 2: Reduced Stress

Being relaxed as you go to bed is like a surgeon showing up stress-free for work: it just makes the tasks at hand easier, thus creating a positive cycle that improves efficiency. Because the task at hand during weight loss is waste elimination, being less stressed is good news.

Stress management and stress reduction are omnipresent issues of our era, so it should be relatively easy for you to find pertinent info on stress management tools, exercise and other such stress-release techniques, schedule balance, changes in mental scenery, regular reassessment of one's life/objectives/priorities, etc. As you will discover in Step 6, we value the impact of stress management on weight loss enough to have included it as one of the six steps of this program.

INTERNAL FACTOR 3: Better Health

Better health begets better sleep. Many individuals will willingly partake in unhealthy activities (e.g., bad diet, alcohol, cigarette, inactivity) and adopt an *"I'll just sleep it off"* attitude. Not a good idea for weight loss, for what you do during waking hours contributes significantly to what occurs during sleeping hours, and vice versa.

INTERNAL FACTOR 4: Empty Stomach

As mentioned earlier, having food in your stomach while sleeping can be disruptive. Our experience has shown that eating food before retiring at night impairs sleep. On top of that, less energy regenerated in totality makes for a more tired body the next day; because toxins are also eliminated during our waking hours, being tired also impairs this process. Over time, toxins accumulate and overweight ensues.

Some of you may actually experience "good" sleep shortly after a meal. That's because you've been going to sleep with food in your stomach for such a long time that you don't really recall sleep ever being better than what it has been and what it is today. It's like anyone who has endured chronic pain for years...they usually only realize how much pain they were enduring the day the pain goes away...until then, the pain was so part of their daily lives that they had become somewhat numb to it. The same goes for sleep: when you manage to retire on an empty stomach for a few consecutive nights, you will be pleasantly surprised at the net improvement of its quality.

INTERNAL FACTOR 5: Relaxed Mindset

If your head is full of stressful thoughts just before retiring at night, these may carry into your deeper sleep and interfere with its quality. Partake in relaxing activities just before falling asleep: read a comic book or a calming novel, listen to soothing music, stretch, do yoga, meditate, do breathing exercises, etc. Let the last thing on your mind be something pleasant as you sink into unconsciousness.

INTERNAL FACTOR 6: Drug-Free Sleep

Drug-induced sleep greatly reduces physical/mental faculties and activities as the body wrestles with the drug, which it considers a nuisance and a poison. Given that most sleep-inducing drugs are pretty powerful, it's like wrestling with a bull: try it and see if it doesn't affect your physical and mental faculties...! As a result, the presence of drugs interferes greatly with toxin elimination.

EXTERNAL FACTOR 1: Fresh Circulating Air

We exhale a toxin called carbon dioxide. If what you breathe out doesn't leave the room because of poor air circulation, then you are likely to breathe some of that CO_2 back in. Open a window and let the air circulate; even if the outside air is polluted, it is better than breathing in your own waste or exudes of anyone else sharing your room.

Are winters cold where you live? No worries. Simply open both bedroom window and door *ever so slightly*, thus creating a current and ensuring that the air you breathe out has a chance to leave the room.

Not only does air circulation reduce your chances of breathing CO_2 back in, but it also contributes to overall better sleep, which in turn contributes to overall better toxin elimination.

The High School Reunion

Rachel opened the letter. It was an invitation to her 20-year high school reunion.

She had been a star runner in high school, twice Athlete of the Year.

Then came the professional and the family life and, next thing you know, she had lost her shape and had gained a lot of weight. Most people saw this as a natural consequence of time, aging, having kids, etc. But Rachel had always been proud of being somewhat of an overachiever, and found it hard to accept how things had become.

She had not gone to her 10-year reunion.

Jamie and Sarah now entered her mind, and how they were starting to put on a little weight. "They're not even 10!" she thought.

Today, Rachel heads the High School Reunion Committee, runs a good 6-7 miles every day, and coaches the local high school track & field team, of which are part both Jamie and Sarah...

EXTERNAL FACTOR 2: Quiet and Dark Surroundings

A noise-free and light-free environment is conducive to better sleep. If there is noise beyond your control, like traffic noise or passing trains, then simply use ear-plugs, or try masking it with a low-level constant soothing one, like playing nature noises (ocean, waterfall, wind, etc.) or relaxing music. If there is lighting beyond your control, wear eye covering. Either way, aim for quiet and dark.

EXTERNAL FACTOR 3: Comfortable Bed and Bedding

A comfortable bed is usually one that offers better weight distribution, like a waterbed or a viscoelastic mattress (as made popular by the brand Tempur-Pedic®). Weight distribution is related to pressure points, meaning those body parts that are in contact with the mattress. The more contact points (or pressure points), the less weight per point, the more comfort, and the better the sleep. Since you spend about one third of life sleeping, a good mattress is worth the investment.

Also, since skin needs proper air circulation at its surface, you'll want to include bedding made up of natural fabrics that "breathe," such as cotton.

EXTERNAL FACTOR 4: A Stress-Free Bed Partner

The human body emanates various energies, like infrared heat, electro-photonic emissions, biophoton emissions and electromagnetic fields. If your bed partner is stressed, then his/her emissions and his/her tossing and turning may disrupt your sleep. We understand you may have very little control over your partner's stress levels, but if you believe there is anything to be done, then it's worth a try. Keep in mind that every lifestyle element you are able to transform gets you one step closer to your weight loss goals.

EXTERNAL FACTOR 5: Adequate Temperature

It's very simple: not too hot and not too cold. We all react differently to ambient temperature, so find the one that is best for you. Adequate temperature may seem trivial, but consider that thermoregulation, even in parsecs, requires a lot of energy...energy that could be better used toward toxin elimination, so give this as much importance as any of the other weight loss components. *"God is in the details,"* as they say...

Quantity

"The amount of sleep required by the average person is five minutes more."

— **Wilson Mizener**
American playwright

The adequate amount of sleep needed to contribute to weight loss is variable from one individual to the next. To establish true sleep needs, you would need to let your body wake up on its own (as opposed to waking up with an alarm clock) for an extended period of time, say, while on vacation. Some of you never use an alarm clock because you've conditioned your body to wake up on its own after a set number of hours; chances are, however that your sleep could use some improvement. Being on vacation would enable you to break this conditioned reflex. If you knew when you fell asleep that you had nothing scheduled the next morning, and the morning after that, and so on, for an extended period of time (say 1-2 months), then your body would eventually transform your poor sleep into very good, deep and recuperative sleep, and find its own *natural* quantity. Ending sleep *prematurely* (with the use of alarm clocks or out of habit) also means ending its elimination cycle prematurely, which is obviously not ideal for weight loss.

Most days, I still set an alarm clock, but only as a safety net. My body needs a naturally healthy sleeping period of approximately six hours (may not seem a lot for most people, but the cleaner your body gets, the less sleep it needs), so I set the alarm seven hours later. This way, I usually wake up much before my alarm ever goes off; the alarm is for peace of mind, in case I were to unexpectedly sleep beyond my usual six hours.

As you begin the weight loss program, you may notice that you need *more* sleep. This is expected, and temporary. The weight loss program enables the body to produce extraordinary waste elimination. Given this rare opportunity to cleanse itself, and not knowing if the situation is to be permanent, your body will take advantage of this situation and work overtime; this accounts for the sudden extra need for sleep. As waste elimination continues, however, toxin levels will decrease. Consequently, your sleep quantity will diminish *naturally*. As your body becomes cleaner, sleep periods will be shorter yet more recuperative!

Here are a few miscellaneous notes to consider:

- Mental workers sleep more than physical workers.
- Working outdoors all day and sleeping outdoors (vs. working indoors and sleeping indoors) decreases sleeping time by 1 to 2 hours per night.
- A less intoxicated body needs less sleep.
- What you do during your waking hours (combined with your past sleeping hours) will determine your future needs for sleep.
- During sleep, two important weight loss phenomena occur: less waste is generated and more waste is expelled.
- Including a few sleep hours before midnight creates better overall recuperation.
- In an ideal world, one would sleep between sunset and sunrise.

To conclude, follow the guidelines establishing good *quality* sleep, and the *quantity* will regulate itself naturally. If at all possible, try to change your schedule so as to get enough sleep before the alarm clock goes off; this way, the alarm only acts as a backup plan should you fail to wake up on your own, which is, as far as I'm concerned, a better start to everyday...

Adequate Sleep Checklist

Dates, from _____ to _____

Simply insert "yes," "no," "N/A" (for "not applicable") in the appropriate cells. Use before your next sleep period.

	Sun	Mon	Tue	Wed	Thu	Fri	Sat
Did I eat well today?							
Did I exercise today?							
Did I keep stress to a minimum?							
Was my day free of smoke, drugs or alcohol?							
Is there good air circulation in my bedroom?							
Is it quiet and dark in my bedroom?							
Is my bed and bedding comfortable?							
Am I going to sleep beside a stress-free partner tonight?							
Is the temperature adequate in my bedroom?							
Will I be going to bed on an empty stomach?							
Do I have a plan to clear my mind before falling asleep?							
Have I gotten rid of my sleeping pills?							
Do I have it set up so that the alarm is plan B, and not plan A?							

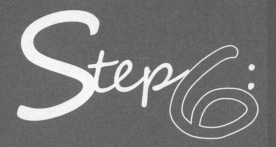

Step 6: Managing Stress to Promote Toxin Elimination

"It is our choices...that show what we truly are, far more than our abilities."

— **J.K. Rowling**
author of *Harry Potter*

"Too many people spend money they haven't earned, to buy things they don't want, to impress people they don't like."

— **Will Smith**

Question: *Does stress cause weight gain?*
Answer: *Yes, in various ways. For example:*

- We tend to eat more ("binge eating") in periods of high stress, and we also reach for "comfort foods" (e.g., chocolate, chips, sweets, coffee, tea, carbonated drinks, tobacco and alcohol), often high in refined sugar and other unhealthy substances.
- Our sleep quality is diminished, and thus the elimination process is hindered.
- Dealing with stress during waking hours requires the body to divert energy and resources from all other ongoing physiological tasks, including toxin elimination.
- Stressful periods produce more internal toxins.

The impact of stress on weight gain is not as significant as that of food, exercise and sleep, but it is real, and knowing this will hopefully produce an added incentive to create a lifestyle that integrates strategic stress management.

If you're driven, then you probably don't think your present stress levels influence your weight in any way. In fact, you are likely tempted to skip this chapter because you don't feel it's pertinent to your situation. Although not impossible, chances that your present stress management is not contributing to your extra weight are very slim.

Consider that we were designed to live in a context of abundance. Today's society is anything but that. Love is scarce. Sex is scarce. Trust is scarce. Safety is scarce. Money is scarce. Downtime is scarce. And all of this scarcity creates stress. From the moment you get up in the morning, there is an unhealthy background stress that permeates your life. Just like most unpleasant elements of life, you have become somewhat numb to it. I'm not referring to more acute or sudden stresses, like avoiding a car accident, finding out that someone has sustained an injury or learning that you have shorter deadlines for a project. No. I'm referring to a more subtle but constant stress, like worrying about health matters, extra weight, your children's safety, financial issues, etc. Similar to the constant humming of a machine, it's there, but you have endured it for so long that you don't pay attention to it anymore...and it affects your health and weight.

My recommendation: assess your present life and get to work on making changes. It may sound simple, but take a close look at your life and you'll see just how much tidying there is to do. Here are a few leads:

1. Identify and Re-Structure Your Stressors.
2. Bring Balance to Your Schedule.
3. Get to Know Thyself.
4. Determine How Long You Want to Sustain Bad Stress.
5. Always Look for New Sources of Motivation.

Identify and Re-Structure Your Stressors

"I believe you make your day. You make your life. So much of it is all perception, and this is the form that I built for myself. I have to accept it and work within those compounds, and it's up to me. "
— **Brad Pitt**

Identify the various stressors in your life, and then re-structure them. Just like a New Year's resolution, it's time to take the pulse on your situation and make some improvements. Begin by identifying:

- Good stressors (e.g., going on a date)
- Bad stressors that are likely to stay (e.g., work)
- Bad stressors that must be resolved at once (e.g., extra weight)

In order to re-structure your life to be less stressful, get to the latter type first. It's illogical to keep doing the dishes if the house is burning, right? If your health and finances are a great source of stress, then you must focus all of your attention on getting these under control *as a priority*. You may already know this, of course, but you've just been putting it off for whatever reasons...time to get to it!

Here's a suggestion: list your stressors, and then proceed to keep the good ones, improve the bad-but-likely-to-stay, and deal with the bad-and-must-be-resolved-at-once. For example:

Good Stressors (to keep)	Bad Stressors (likely to stay)	Bad Stressors (must be resolved at once)
Going on a date	Work	Extra weight
About to perform a show or compete in sports	Air & noise pollution	Financial debt
Building a new home	Income tax	Unresolved issues with loved ones
Bikini season just around the corner	Commute to work	Working overtime

Do this re-structuring process quickly and efficiently. For example, don't lay out a long-term plan to get your finances under control. The longer you give yourself to achieve a result, the fewer chances you have of getting it done...motivation will wean down, and various reasons to procrastinate will surface.

Just imagine...how much lighter and more fun life would be if you resolved, say, even just 1 major issue? How would things be different? Imagine if you licked 3 or 4 of these important issues...how would your spirits be then?

Bring Balance to Your Schedule

"When I get logical, and I don't trust my instincts...that's when I get in trouble."

— Angelina Jolie

I like visual representations, and so I like to look at my life through colored schedules, graphs and charts. This way, it's easier to spot the imbalances. I often look at my schedules from all angles (e.g., daily, weekly, monthly and yearly).

Last year, for example, my stress levels were a little too elevated, so I decided to get a clear image of my life to really see where I was investing my time and energy. I began by listing all activities that made up a typical week and their duration. I then divided the amount of time allotted to each activity by total weekly hours (168) in order to obtain percentages and build nice charts. It was important not to get stuck trying to account for every minute of every day; however, it was also important not to omit what may have seemed trivial (e.g., the amount of time spent getting from one place to the next while running errands and commuting) but was in fact very time consuming when totaled.

My weekly life a year ago (percentages have been rounded off):

- **Eat:** 30 minutes per meal x 3 meals per day x 7 days = 11 hours or 7% of my total week
- **Exercise:** 5h per week or 3%
- **Getting from one place to the next** (ex. commute, going to the movies): 19h or 11%
- **House chores and errands** (ex. house cleaning, laundry, grocery shopping): 7h or 4%
- **Human warmth and touch** (ex. massage, sex, intimacy): 3h or 2%
- **Personal hygiene and grooming** (ex. shower, shave, haircut, brush teeth): 5h or 3%
- **Sleep:** 8 hours per day x 7 days = 56h or 33%
- **Social** (ex. party, drinks with friends, dancing) **and entertainment** (ex. movie, concert): 6h or 4%
- **Work:** 56h or 33%

My weekly life today:

- **Eat:** 1 hour per meal x 3 meals per day x 7 days = 21h or 13%
- **Exercise:** 1 hour per day x 7 days = 7 hours or 4% of my total week
- **Getting from one place to the next:** 14h or 8%
- **House chores and errands:** 3h or 2%
- **Human warmth and touch:** 14h or 8%
- **Leisure** (ex. read a book, walk in the park): 8h or 5%
- **Personal hygiene and grooming:** 5h or 3%
- **Sleep:** a little under 6 hours per day x 7 days = 41h or 24%
- **Social and entertainment:** 27h or 16%
- **Work:** 28h or 17%

Which, as pie charts, looks something like this:

My Weekly Life a Year Ago

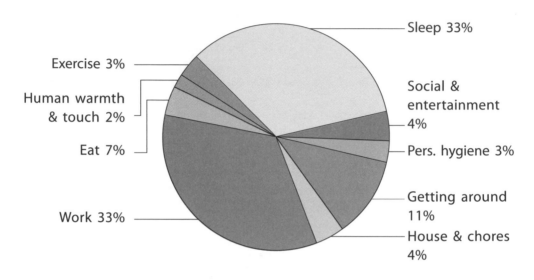

Sleep 33%

Exercise 3%

Human warmth & touch 2%

Social & entertainment 4%

Eat 7%

Pers. hygiene 3%

Getting around 11%

Work 33%

House & chores 4%

My Weekly Life Today

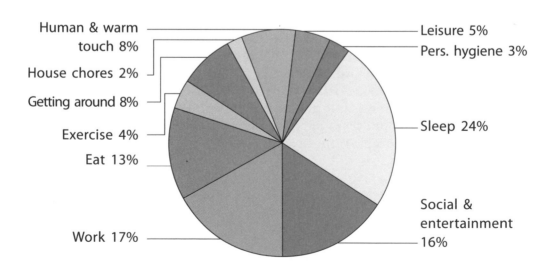

Human & warm touch 8%

Leisure 5%

Pers. hygiene 3%

House chores 2%

Getting around 8%

Exercise 4%

Sleep 24%

Eat 13%

Work 17%

Social & entertainment 16%

Today I sleep less, yet I'm better rested. I work less, yet my financial situation has improved. My "social & entertainment" category has brought me more variety and more fun. I now have a "leisure" category. I have changed my exercise habits to be more in the great outdoors, which has brought me more natural stimulation (just so you know, trapped indoor air and artificial lighting is not the best). I spend much more time doing pleasant things rather than just going from one place to the next doing unpleasant and unfulfilling things. Generally, my stress levels have gone down, my energy has gone up, and because my schedule is more balanced, I am much happier.

For anyone trying to lose weight, this is good news.

Get to Know Thyself

"I've finally stopped running away from myself. Who else is there better to be? "

— **Goldie Hawn**

Making the right choices is not always easy. Having life issues that just never seem to get resolved can be very disempowering and frustrating. Not understanding others can lead to confusion and irritation.

Knowing yourself better can give you a great deal of power with such matters.

I'm not suggesting you go looking for problems that aren't really there; if you're a regular happy-go-lucky person, then you may not feel you have any personal self-inquiry to do. If, however, you feel that some issues could have been dealt with a long time ago, and you know you have just been sweeping them under the rug, then I suggest you get to them as quickly as possible. The average adult is made up of 75 to 125 trillion cells...carrying the weight of unresolved issues on your shoulders impairs their proper function, which consequently produces additional toxins and impairs waste elimination.

If you're interested in any type of self-improvement or personal growth medium and don't know where to start, here's something I highly recommend: www.landmarkeducation.com.

Resolving issues may not have as quick or as visible an impact on weight loss as food and exercise but, over time, it does make a difference.

To illustrate, imagine all the weight-promoting elements of your lifestyle (e.g., improperly combined meals, sedentary activities, unresolved issues and poor sleep) as pebbles, and your ideal weight as a glass window; the more pebbles are thrown against the glass, the higher the chances of it breaking. The opposite is also true, of course: fewer pebbles means lower risk of window break.

Determine How Long You Want to Sustain Bad Stress

"Insanity: doing the same thing over and over again and expecting different results."

— **Albert Einstein**

Stress was designed to be short-lived, a few minutes at most, like the time needed to fight or flee a predator. Sustaining stress beyond this time (e.g., being preoccupied with extra weight, worrying about finances 24/7, stressing about losing your job) is very unhealthy and, believe it or not, contributes to weight gain.

As you live your various stresses, train yourself to recognize when a healthy stress period is about to become unhealthy, and then find ways to reduce this unhealthy stress time. For example, working at a computer less than 2 hours is still an OK stress for me, but if I push beyond that, it starts to become a bad stress...my focus weans, my body begins to ache, it's difficult to find a comfortable position, my eyes become tired and dry, etc.

Here are a few other personal examples:

- Spending more than 10 minutes thinking about tomorrow's issues as I go to bed. The reason I'm in bed in the first place is to fall asleep, not to focus on next days' worries.
- Feuding for more than 5 minutes after an argument with loved ones. Often, I would like to be silently righteous for as long as possible (in moments of anger, being right just feels gooood...), but the people I care for are too important to let pride and righteousness dictate my way of being.

- More than 1 day of knowing I should have already exercised. I usually exercise in the morning so, once it's done, it's done. If I do not exercise in the morning, then I start to worry about it until I get to it. Noon hits, I'm thinking about it. Mid-afternoon comes around, my guilt increases. Evening arrives and now I don't even have the motivation to do it, so I put it behind me and start to plan for tomorrow. If I were to keep carrying the guilt all evening and all night, and wake up the next morning still preoccupied about not having exercised the day before, then it would have become unhealthy stress.

It is not always necessary to chronologically define the limit between the healthy and unhealthy zones. In other words, we do not need to establish a precise time; if we listen to our bodies, we know when we have gone beyond a good stress period and that something needs to be done. We don't need to look at our watch, because we just know.

Mall Santa

"It's like getting hit by a train," was Rick's first thought...

"But I'm only 52," was his second...

Rick was a successful self-made businessman. He had put 2 kids through college. He was a Little League Coach every summer and a Mall Santa every Christmas. Most free weekends were spent fly-fishing with lifelong friends.

"You had double bypass surgery, Mr. Douglas," the doctor told him.

Rick knew he would have to lose weight.

And he did. It wasn't easy and, for almost 2 years, he harped at it, but in the end, managed to lose 100 lbs.

It's been 15 years since the heart attack. Not a day goes by that Rick doesn't think that he's never loved life so much, and that he's never lived it so fully. *"There's no way I wasn't going to be around to cash in on my pension,"* he often tells his buddies...

"And there's no way I wasn't going to be around to see my grandchildren grow up," he often tells his wife.

Always Look for New Sources of Motivation

"Excitement is the more practical synonym for happiness, and it is precisely what you should strive to chase. It is the cure-all."
— **Timothy Ferriss**
best-selling author of *The 4-Hour Work Week*

From the time you get out of bed in the morning to the moment you go to sleep at night, life doesn't naturally throw exciting and motivating things your way. The sad reality of today's society is that exciting and motivating moments are scarce, so you have to perpetually find new ways to create them yourself...or else projects and dreams have but little chance of ever seeing the light of day. In other words, you will have to *generate* motivation because it is not going to happen by itself.

Although you probably already knew this, it's important you consider it newly. If you find yourself *wanting* to go forth with a project (like losing weight) but find *no motivation*, look for sources that will make a difference. It could be a conversation with a friend, a book, a seminar, an inspiring movie or You Tube videos of motivational speakers (e.g., Anthony Robbins, Jack Canfield and Bob Proctor); or, as mentioned in Step 2 (Dream List), having exciting things in your schedule. Dropping money into a savings account, for example, is not an exciting activity, but the vacation that's possible with those funds is. Getting ready for a night on the town stirs up excitement, not because fixing your hair and putting on make-up is overly titillating, but rather because you already see yourself with friends on the dance floor. Same goes for weight loss...you need to identify *what will be possible* with a new slim and fit body. If things are to move forward, there needs to be a carrot in front of the horse.

On a last note, consider that you get in life what you have the courage to ask for, and that there's no Mama Bird to push you out of the nest.

Stress Management
Checklist

Simply insert "yes," "no," "N/A" (for "not applicable") or date & time in the appropriate cells.

	Done	Not done yet, but will be done by... (insert time & date, then make a promise to a friend that it will be done by established time & date, and then call him/her when it's done)
Have I identified and restructured my stressors?		
Have I reworked my schedule?		
Do I have a plan for self-exploration and personal growth?		
Have I identified time periods for sustaining various bad stresses?		
Have I found new sources of motivation?		

Life After This Book

"The future depends on what we do in the present."
— **Gandhi**

"In questions of science, the authority of a thousand is not worth the humble reasoning of a single individual."
— **Galileo**

Congratulations, you have completed the theoretical part of your program. It is the first step in your weight loss adventure. The next step, of course, is putting all this new information and these new guidelines into practice. This is the most important step, for you will not lose weight by simply reading a book.

As stated previously, please note that "putting the book's guidelines into practice" doesn't mean that you have to apply these 100% overnight. Great if you can, but no stress if you can't. The success of the weight loss program does not depend on its *full application*; in other words, it is possible to lose weight even by just applying *some* of the information contained herein. The more you do it, of course, the better the chances of success.

Moreover, integrating this program is similar to learning a new sport or starting a new job...being good at it may require some time. Same here: apply the guidelines progressively and you will start to see results; aim to apply more and more of these guidelines, and you will become better at losing weight and see even more results.

In Part 2, we have included succulent recipes for individuals who like to spend time in the kitchen, and tricks for those who like to eat out.

Being Lean and Fit in a Weight-Promoting World

"If you can't beat them, arrange to have them beaten."
— **George Carlin**

Question: *"Is it easy being lean and fit in a weight-promoting world?"*
Answer: *Well, it may not be easy...*

Food and nutrition today are complicated, confusing, unhealthy yet very powerfully addictive. The food industry invests billions of dollars every year to make sure you ingest their products and, believe you me, they have it down to a science! Every detail is carefully and strategically planned...marketing colors, packaging design, super athlete sponsors, eye-level product placement, sampling tables, grocery cart size to promote purchasing, trendy TV commercials, flashy roadside signs, catchy tunes, etc., etc., etc. It's difficult to remain immune to this insidious marketing.

Fending off the food industry sharks is one thing, but we also have to realize just how much we're making it hard on ourselves. Firstly, by making food our solution to unfulfilled stimulation (how often do we eat to reward ourselves?)...and then, by eating out of habit, and not necessarily out of hunger (e.g., while driving, watching TV or reading the newspaper) and even worse, by using food as an excuse to create and structure social events (e.g., business meetings, family gatherings or evenings out with friends) evidently, dealing with such self-destructive patterns can be very exhausting.

Food is one thing, but what about other lifestyle components? Will incorporating these be easy? Well, you'll be swimming against the current once more. If you don't schedule exercise, you'll end up having spent your entire week sitting somewhere: in front of the TV, at a computer, in a car, etc. Unless you put some effort into changing your sleeping conditions, you're likely to become one of the million individuals who suffer from any of the hundreds of sleeping disorders known today. And, last but not least, if you refuse to see the true impact of stress on your life and don't get around to changing a few things, then you are definitely in for an unpleasant surprise.

So society won't make it easy for you.

Moreover, you'll find yourself dealing with social prejudice (e.g., being labeled as bizarre with your new lifestyle) and isolation (e.g., not many others around you eating the way you do). Self-doubt may creep in and your own social conditioning of many years will prove to be the biggest obstacle of all.

So no, being lean and fit may not be easy...

BUT IT IS POSSIBLE, and the good news is that *you* are in charge. Only you get to say whether or not you lose weight. No one else will, so you can either stay on the social weight-promoting roller coaster (and suffer the pathological consequences) or you can take charge of your own fate and produce desired results. We did, and we love food just as the next person. We partake in many sedentary activities. We deal with every-day stress just like you do. But, at the end of the day, we manage to create a lifestyle as outlined in this book, which gives us our ideal healthy weight. On the front cover photography, David is 39 and I am 28; we have never felt better and only feel like we're getting younger.

If lifestyle changes seem long and arduous, and fill you with hesitation or discouragement, consider that today's *few* extra pounds may very quickly become tomorrow's *many* extra pounds, and being overweight is a concern that goes beyond looks and can be very hazardous to one's health. It is linked as a risk factor in cardiovascular disease, high-blood pressure, lung disease, respiratory problems, arthritis, osteoarthritis, varicose veins, non-insulin-dependent diabetes mellitus (type II), gallbladder disease, certain cancers (colon, breast and uterus) and sleep apnea.

If you're still unsure about when to be in action, then answer the following question and see where it takes you...

"How would my life be different if I lost those extra pounds?"

Go now, dream and take the next step.

David & Helene

Part 2

By Helene

"Many of the truths we cling to depend greatly on our own point of view.."

— **Obi-Wan-Kenobi**
Star Wars: Return of the Jedi

Before We Step into the Kitchen

"I was 32 when I started cooking; up until then, I just ate."
— **Julia Child**

"I eat too much because I'm depressed, and I'm depressed because I eat too much. It's a vicious circle...that took years to perfect!"
— **Garfield the cat**

Welcome to my world: FOOD! Mmm...eating...soooo much fun, isn't it? From age 17, I pursued a goal to find and create both *tasty* and *healthy* meals. I read books on healthy eating. I studied and worked in the food and service industry as a waitress and as a sommelier. I spent a lot of time in restaurant kitchens, learning from chefs as they prepared succulent meals. Five years into this quest, I had found many *tasty* meals, but none that were simultaneously *healthy*. Then I met David and discovered what healthy eating really was. Tasty AND healthy was finally possible...

Y ou may be under the impression that eating according to the principles of Step 3 makes things more complicated for someone who likes to prepare food. Well, we have found just the opposite. Think about it: fewer ingredients, less cooking and practically no dirty dishes...doesn't get much simpler than that, now does it? For you kitchen wizards, our recipes will be a "piece of cake," so to speak. For you novices, do not fear, because here's the thing to know: *making truly healthy recipes is much easier and faster than making ill-combined meals.* Not as simple as microwaving frozen dinners or using store-made spaghetti sauce mind you, but still pretty easy, much tastier and much healthier.

On another note, as mentioned in Step 3, the Recommended Eating Guidelines were elaborated as "something to aim for," and not as "a discipline hammer with which to hit yourself every time you're not respecting their application." Although it is possible to respect these guidelines 100%, it is not necessary in order to produce weight loss. Even we, as authors of this book, are not "purists": we eat in a way to keep the weight off, but to also enjoy ourselves. Moreover, you will notice that some of the recipes in Part 2 come in contradiction with certain Recommended Eating Guidelines...it's OK...we've created them to still produce weight loss. The idea behind the Guidelines is that everyone, from extremely disciplined to a little bit less disciplined, can find what works for them.

To help you along, we've added approximate gastric evacuation times. *Again, these times are approximations and may vary from one individual to the next, and may also vary if factors such as fatigue, stress, meal size, alcohol, etc., are present.* The longer you give your digestive system to deal with the last meal, the better the chances of losing weight.

In addition, we have created common recipes, like pizzas and burgers; don't expect the *exact* same taste as popular pizzas and burgers, because we have adapted them to promote weight loss, but expect them to be very tasty nonetheless. Use the information from Step 3 to determine what's healthy, and then include the following tips to create something sinfully delicious:

1. Use high-quality ingredients...and *some* condiments and spices.
2. Don't be a slave to measurements...taste and adjust as you prepare.

Use High-Quality Ingredients...and Some Condiments and Spices

There are many ways to prepare a tasty meal, some of which are:

1. Using *only* high-quality ingredients.
2. Using high-quality ingredients and adding *some* condiments and spices.
3. Using low-quality ingredients and adding *many* condiments and spices.
4. Using high-quality ingredients and adding *many* condiments and spices.

Out of those options, however, only two promote weight loss. Yes, you've guessed it, numbers 1 and 2. There are a great many savory meals to be found in today's society, but unfortunately most of them are weight-promoting. The good news is that it is very possible and very simple to prepare both savory *and* healthy meals. It begins by finding high-quality ingredients.

Choosing Your Ingredients

Your chances of finding high-quality ingredients will greatly increase if you shop at your local market place, health-food stores and specialty/import grocery boutiques. It is not to say that you cannot find any high-quality ingredients in larger surface food stores, but these usually offer the blander highly processed varieties. Fruits and vegetables, for example, tend to be unripe, waxed, irradiated, tasteless and covered in hazardous food preservatives. Since the name of the game is both "tasty" and "healthy," start exploring outside the more conventional larger surface food stores.

When purchasing produce, I invite you to:

- **Ask Vendors for Their Opinion.**

  They usually know what's fresh and what's "in season." Buying produce when "in season" ensures variety and freshness.

- **Be Adventurous and Try New Produce.**

  There are over a thousand varieties of eatable fruits and vegetables... how many have you tried? Don't let unfamiliarity stop you from trying new foods or recipes. There is a whole universe of healthy gustatory pleasures to be discovered out there.

- **Train Yourself to Better Select.**

  Use the Web and other sources to get information on how to determine ripeness specific to those fruits and vegetables of your liking. Whole watermelon, for example, is usually odorless, but may still be ripe; look for the ones already cut, or ask if you can sample. Honeydew and cantaloupe on the other hand, will be aromatic when ready.

  Also, when purchasing dried fruits or vegetables, look for those without preservative agents. Dried fruits, for example, are often covered with vegetable oil or sulfites. Look for the items with no other ingredients but the items themselves on the ingredients list: dried figs should read "ingredients: fig" only, and nothing else.

"Health" or "Organic" Sections

When grocery shopping, always remember to check the "Health" or "Organic" sections of your local food store. As mentioned in Step 3, fewer toxins are likely to accumulate in the body if foods have fewer ingredients. Breads, crackers and pasta, for example, should be made with "integral" flour (as opposed to "refined" or all-purpose flour), a few other ingredients (aim for no more than water, yeast, sourdough, vegetable oil, salt, herbs and spices) but nothing weight-promoting (e.g., sugar, eggs, vinegar, dairy products or any bizarre-looking chemical compound). As another example, look for dairy substitutes such as beverages made from soy, rice, almond or oat, cheese-like items made from vegetable oils, etc.

Although not every product in the "Health" or "Organic" sections is healthy and adequate for weight loss (in fact, many are not), *some* may still be found. To choose wisely, simply follow the guidelines as outlined in Step 3 and in this chapter.

A Word on "Organic"

Consumers beware! The word "organic" is sometimes misused:

- in order to be trendy and sell more product, or
- because, given that the standardizing organizations (e.g., FDA and USDA) do not always have enough resources to properly control the certification process, the quality has gone unchecked, or
- with bigger corporations creating their own certification bodies, quality control becomes biased.

As far as I'm concerned, "organic" should only be used when produce has been grown, transformed and prepared naturally, without the use of pesticides, herbicides, fungicides, preservatives or chemical additives of any kind, and, especially, has not been genetically altered. For example, say you sample from 3 different bags of carrots at your local grocery store:

1. The first one is not labelled "organic"; its price is 2$ and the carrots, well, they're all identical, watery tasting and so orange that they probably glow in the dark.

2. The second bag is $3, from a small local farmer (as you notice from the name and address on the bag); its carrots are all irregular-sized, look a little unwashed (hints of soil in the folds), but are crunchy and tasty.

3. The third bag is labelled "organic" and costs $5; the carrots look clean and somewhat identical; the taste has a little something pungent to it (like pesticide pungent).Well, you've guessed it: the only real "organic" carrots would be no.2. Training yourself to differentiate healthy foods from unhealthy foods is an exercise in freethinking, for you have to break from the conditioning of the past. Buying from local growers and farmers is usually a good start to finding true "organic" products.

When you read "vegetable oil" in our recipes, you are free to choose any one of the following (CAPITALIZED being much more aromatic). Select *extra virgin first cold press* oils for higher nutrient value:

Avocado	GRILLED SESAME	Safflower
Canola	HAZELNUT	Sesame
COCONUT	Olive	Soy
Corn	Palm	Sunflower
Cotton seed	Peanut	TRUFFLE
Flax seed	PISTACHIO	WALNUT

For other oiling components (or for spreading purposes), here are a few suggestions:

- puréed or mashed avocado
- butter
- vegetable oil spread (olive, coconut, canola)

Stay away from hydrogenated products, like margarine, as these are very hard to digest and only end up adding to the toxic load. There are healthier products out there, like Solid Olive for example (from France, www.solidolive.com, imported regularly to North America by www.tribeca-imports.com).

Mayonnaise

This condiment is widely used in today's society. The chemical nature of its ingredients (egg yolks, vinegar, etc.), however, makes it weight-promoting. For healthier alternatives, look for the "no eggs, no dairy" varieties.

My favourite, because it surprisingly tastes like the "real" thing: *Vegenaise* from *Earth Island Natural Food* (www.followyourheart.com).

Salt, herbs and spices fall into the "irritants" category (as seen in Guideline no.14). They are highly stimulating and intensify flavors, but are toxic and thus contribute to weight gain. This said, I do use salt, herbs and spices, *but very sparingly.* Because flavor enhancers are so omnipresent, our tongue has been used to their very intense stimulation; it's time to break from this conditioning. Like primary colors, there are primary gustatory sensations: sweet, sour, acid and bitter. Just like colors, however, there are many mixes and blends of these tastes, giving way to a host of gustatory "shades." As you begin to reduce the use of irritants, your tongue will set a new standard of taste by default, and you will rediscover the richness of flavors of foods' natural composition. Much like a wine can be described by the soil in which its grapes have grown (called a *terroir)*, so can fruits and vegetables if your tongue is given a break from flavor enhancers. An apple may have hints of honey, mint and violets; celery may be sweet or acrid; bananas may have aromas of vanilla or cinnamon; etc. In time, your tongue will learn to pick up on these gustatory "shades." Eating healthier re-trains your taste buds to appreciate the naturally present softer, fuller and richer flavors of food, so there's less need to add anything strong.

You will also notice in the recipe section that some ingredients, like *vegetable oil, sea salt and freshly squeezed lemon juice,* are used frequently. This is done to add value or to bring balance, but not to overshadow the taste of the main ingredients. Basically, salt enhances flavors (even the sweet ones), while lemon or lime juice brings acidity to balance a bland meal. Oily agents, on the other hand, capture and bring out aromas, and link the various textures of a meal. So add these ingredients, initially in small quantities, then taste, adjust, and add more if need be. Ideally, recipes should taste like the main ingredients and not like the flavor enhancers.

Salt

There are many forms of salt out there: unrefined (such as sea salt), refined and iodized. Unrefined is better. Sea salt comes in table-sized or bigger crystals (used in a salt grinder). My favorite is "fleur de sel" (from the French, literally "flower of salt"), which is a hand-harvested sea salt; expensive, but most definitely worth it.

In regards to herbs, know that dried herbs are usually more flavorful than their fresh equivalent. If you want to use dried herbs instead of fresh ones, apply a 1 to 3 ratio; 2 oz. of dried parsley, for example, would be equal to 6 oz. of fresh parsley.

Dried herbs are excellent for longer cooking (e.g., hot soups). Buy small quantities and store them for *short periods*, for they dry and lose their flavors rapidly; if you've had dried herbs sitting in your cupboards for more than a year, please throw them out. Dried herbs are good for use when their green color is not yet faded and when their aromas are still strong (test by crushing a few leaves in the palm of your hand and then by smelling).

Fresh herbs, on the other hand, don't keep as long but are just as interesting. Because nothing has been transformed through the dehydration process, their flavors are different than dried herbs... maybe

not as intense, but fuller and well rounded. If you have a green thumb, plant some in your garden (or, for city dwellers, in a flower box on a balcony); this way, you may grow your favorite (mine being basil, thyme, oregano, mint, rosemary and cilantro) and use them for spur-of-the-moment creativity. If you're not inclined to grow fresh herbs, then look for them at your local market; they are very inexpensive and, even at a minimum buy of 1$, I always have too much and end up giving some to my friends and neighbors.

Just to give you an idea, here is a partial list of herbs and spices:

HERBS

Angelica	Cilantro	Marjoram	Savory
Basil	Curry	Mint	Sorrel
Bay leaf	Dill	Oregano	Tarragon
Chervil	Hyssop	Parsley	Thyme
Chives	Lavender	Rosemary	Woodruff
Cicely	Lemongrass	Sage	

SPICES

Allspice	Coriander	Mustard	Sesame
Anise	Cumin	Nutmeg	Sumac
Caraway	Fennel	Paprika	Tamarind
Cardamom	Garlic	Pepper	Turmeric
Chili	Ginger	Poppy seed	Vanilla
Cinnamon	Juniper berry	Saffron	
Cloves	Liquorice	Sarsaparilla	

Don't Be a Slave to Measurements... Taste and Adjust As You Prepare

As you prepare recipes, know that using precise measurements (i.e., 1 oz. of this, a table spoon of that, 8 pieces of this makes 4 portions of that, etc.) *will not guarantee an anticipated result, but your taste buds will.* For example: today you're making a new tomato soup recipe. It's your first time so you follow the instructions very carefully. If you do not taste and adjust as you go along, well, the end product will be a result of chance...maybe it'll be to your liking, maybe it won't...you'll only know when you sit down and eat it. Let's say that, on this particular day, the Gods were in your favor and the soup was exactly how you wanted it to be. In fact, you are so proud of your result you decide to do it again the following week. So here you are, once more, carefully measuring and timing everything in accordance to the written recipe...but the result is surprisingly very different than last time! *"How can that be?"* you ponder, *"I followed the instructions exactly as the previous attempt..."* Well, it's important to know that a given recipe, from one time to the next, may vary because:

- Although the ingredients are the same, their taste is not quite identical—today's tomato may not taste like tomorrow's tomato.
- Mixing or cooking conditions, although seemingly identical, may have varied just enough to change the outcome.
- Etc.

I prepare recipes from motivation and memory, and I adjust by tasting frequently as I prepare. I also like to improvise and use up whatever's lying around so as to limit waste...maybe the original recipe didn't call for that cucumber, but it was sitting in my fridge and very ripe, so I threw it in.

This said, I also strongly encourage you to create recipes according to *your* taste; don't stress yourself by trying to always "do it right." If an obstacle comes your way, like a new recipe that sounded succulent initially (e.g., avocado and saffron sorbet), but came out pretty bland, well, improvise and adapt it to your liking (e.g., adding a little pepper and lemon juice to the sorbet to create balance). There is no recipe police, and you are allowed to do whatever you like.

If you're a novice in the kitchen, however, or if you are preparing given recipes for the first time, I do recommend you take a few notes so you can perfect these creations over time.

The point is, once again, that if you want to be sure of the end product, don't rely *only* on what's written down...taste and adjust as you prepare.

Beauty Is in Simplicity

"Simplicity is the ultimate sophistication."
— **Leonardo Da Vinci**

The food guidelines and the recipes we suggest were created to simplify your eating experience, using the least amount of ingredients to create the most amount of taste. Simplifying has its advantages:

- **It Is Healthier.**

Remember from Step 3, on proper food combining: too many different ingredients risk causing poor digestion.

- **It Makes You Discover New Flavors.**

By reducing the use of ingredients and seasoning agents, you will rediscover the natural taste of food...what do cucumbers taste like without salt? Tomatoes without mayonnaise? Salads topped with a little grilled sesame oil instead of Ranch dressing?

- **It Is Less Time and Energy Consuming.**

Less food preparation usually means less energy used, more money saved and, especially important, less dishes to wash!

As you will note in the recipe descriptions, I seldom specify portions and preparation times, for these vary too much from one individual's appetite to the next, and also from one's cooking techniques and kitchen appliances to the next.

A Few Last Things...

There are 2 lists of recipes on the following pages, one made *according to food type* (protein, fats/oils, starchy foods, etc.) and the other *according to popular divisions* (soups, salads, pasta, etc.). Even though a recipe may include various food types, it is classified under one type only, in regard to the items with the longer gastric evacuation time or the food type present in greater amounts. For example, a recipe with asparagus, pine nuts and truffle oil is listed under "protein" on account of nuts having the longer gastric evacuation time.

Please note that recipes for both lists are the same; they are simply listed differently, on one end to help you with your Recommended Eating Guidelines, and on the other to help you better plan your meals.

Following these lists, in the recipe descriptions, ingredients are in **bold italic**. If they appear more than once in the same recipe, then you'll see them in regular font. This way, you can get an idea of what's needed at a quick glance.

Immediately following these recipes, you will find a cooking glossary.

Enter the recipe section, trust your instincts and "Bon appétit!"

List of Recipes

(According to Food Types)

NON-STARCHY VEGETABLES

ACID FOODS

FRUITS

List of Recipes

(Popular Listing)

SANDWICHES

VARIED DISHES

PASTA

FOR CARNIVORES

Recipes: Fruits

Fruits are the perfect food. They are beautiful in color, design and texture. They smell and taste delicious. They possess all the nutrients we need: water, sugar, amino acids, vitamins, minerals and fatty acids. And they require no preparation...just grab and eat!

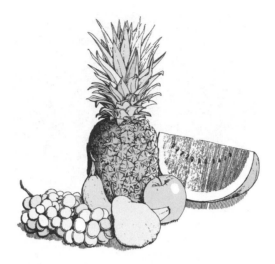

If you're looking for a little variety, however, I suggest using a blender, a juicer or an extractor to make juice or purée. Here are a few suggestions for the blender (unless otherwise specified):

- Liquefy various melon combinations. My favorites are: *watermelon* by itself, *Canary* by itself, or half *cantaloupe* with half *honeydew*.

- *Pineapple* by itself or half pineapple with juice of 2−3 freshly squeezed *oranges* (made with citrus juicer separately).

- 2 *bananas* with 6 Medjol *dates* or 8 Barhi dates. Add 3−8 oz. (89-237 ml) of water to increase fluidity.

- An assortment of *wild berries*, like blueberries, raspberries, strawberries and blackberries.

- Freshly squeezed juice made with citrus juicer): 1 *pink grapefruit* with 4 *honey tangerines*.

- *Apple* and *celery* (even with celery, this is to be considered as a fresh fruit meal for digestive purposes). Make with juice extractor.

- *Mangoes* make great purée. All varieties may be mixed. Here are a few: Haden (most common), Tommy, Kent, Atulfo (yellow, very smooth and creamy) and Francis (also called Haitian mango—very fibrous, sweet and juicy).

- 1 *mango* with 2 *peaches* or 3–4 *apricots*.

- 2 *bananas* and 2 *mangoes*.

- 1 *banana*, 2 *white nectarines*, 1 *mango*.

- 1 *mango* with 10–12 *strawberries*.

Approximate gastric evacuation time for liquid juices, like watermelon or citrus combinations: 30 minutes.

Approximate gastric evacuation time for thicker concoctions, like puréed bananas with dates: 1 hour. Sweet fruits usually take more than 1 hour, but the fact that they are puréed accelerates the passage from the stomach to the small intestine.

Recipes: Cold Soups

Cold soups are great because they are refreshing, easy to prepare and full of nutrients. As part of a starchy meal, all soups may be served with crackers (e.g., www.ryvita.com) or lightly toasted bread.

If soups are made with any vegetables other than avocado, calculate approximately 3 hours of gastric evacuation time; add bread or crackers, then count 4 hours. For soups with avocado, count 4 hours; add bread or crackers, then count 5 hours. Puréed vegetables have a quicker transit time in the stomach. Vegetable oils, although listed in the 4 hour fats/oils category, also have a quicker transit time because of their liquid form. Low-water content starchy foods such as crackers, however, increase the time food is held up in the stomach.

Cream of Avocado

Because avocados tend to oxidize and become brownish rapidly, it is better not to prepare this recipe too much in advance.

In a blender, purée the following ingredients:

- *1 ripe avocado*
- *1 cup of vegetable broth* (add according to desired consistency)
- *Freshly squeezed lemon juice*
- *Sea salt*

Add either ***freshly crushed coriander seeds*** (don't presume they will get crushed in the blender...they usually don't, so crush manually) or ***saffron***.

The avocado and spice (coriander or saffron) should be predominant in taste. In order to achieve this, choose a blander vegetable broth that would not overshadow their flavor. Adjust by adding a little of each ingredients at a time, until you obtain what YOU like.

Mojito Soup

In a blender, purée the following:

- *1 peeled English cucumber* (must be seedless)
- *Juice of half lime* (freshly squeezed)
- *Approx. 15 leaves of fresh mint*
- *Half ripe avocado*
- *Sea salt*
- *1 tablespoon of maple syrup*

Taste to make sure you like the balance between sweet and salty, and enjoy served in a martini glass on a hot summer day as you sit by the pool!

Sweet Bell Pepper Gazpacho

Originally from Spain, the Gazpacho (meaning *remainders* or *worthless things)* is a chilled soup, usually made with olive oil, garlic, stale bread, chopped tomatoes, cucumbers, onions, peppers and herbs. Here's our sweet bell pepper version. In a blender, purée **red**, **orange** and/or **yellow bell peppers** with **olive oil** and **sea salt**. As an option, you may also add either or both **fresh basil** and **sun-dried tomatoes**.

Tomato Gazpacho

In a blender, purée **sweet tomatoes** with **olive oil** and **sea salt**. As an option, you may also add either or both **fresh basil** and **sun-dried tomatoes**.

> **More on the Tomato**
>
> There are more than 100 varieties of tomatoes, with different shapes, colors and taste. When I list sweet tomatoes in recipes, I'm referring to grape tomatoes, cherry tomatoes, yellow and orange tomatoes (any size) or the ones labeled "low acid". You will notice that I sometimes include them in starchy meals...although not ideal, it serves our weight loss goal. When it comes to protein meals, I list more acidic tomatoes, like common pink, red or plum varieties.

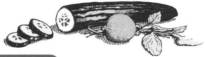

Traditional Gazpacho

- *Fresh sweet tomatoes*
- *Sweet bell peppers*
- *Peeled cucumber*
- *Olive oil*
- *Sea salt*
- *Freshly ground coriander seeds*
- *Freshly ground pepper*
- *Fresh herbs* (basil, oregano, thyme)

In a blender, purée vegetable quantities to end up with 50% tomato, 25% sweet bell pepper and 25% cucumber.

Then, add all other ingredients according to taste. You may also add minced **onion** and, to make it a little more refreshing, **freshly squeeze lemon juice**. Make sure everything is well blended.

Recipes: Hot Soups

Because hot soups taste just as good when re-heated, I suggest you prepare larger batches.

For all soups in this section, count approximately 4 hours of gastric evacuation time. If accompanied with bread or crackers, count 5 hours. Combining many low-water content foods (like bread and crackers) slows gastric evacuation.

Cream of Butternut Squash with Vanilla

- *Butternut squash*
- *Vanilla bean*
- *Vegetable broth*
- *Butter*

Cut Butternut squash in half (lengthwise). Cover cut side with aluminum foil. Place in cooking pan, aluminum side facing up. Cook in oven at 400 °F. Check regularly by piercing flesh with a fork. Cooking time is approximately 40 minutes, but will vary according to squash size. Cooking is done when your fork digs in easily.

While squash is cooking, infuse half a vanilla bean in vegetable broth in a cooking pot for 15−20 minutes. Then, cut open vanilla bean lengthwise and scrape the inside in order to add to broth.

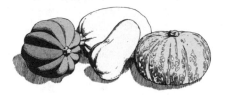

When squash is cooked, remove flesh with a spoon, leaving out the outer layer and its seeds. Mix in with the infused broth in cooking pot. Adjust consistency by adding more vegetable broth or water, and simmer for 1 hour.

Next, remove from heat and add butter while mixing with a fork, creating a smooth texture, and serve.

Note that it is possible to transform this soup to a purée by reducing amount of vegetable broth (used to infuse the vanilla) to a *very small quantity*. You may also vary the recipe by swapping vanilla for nutmeg (no infusion if you do this, of course).

Cream of Carrot & Coconut

- *2 lb of carrots*
- *34 oz. (1 L) vegetable broth*
- *Coconut milk*

Place chopped carrots in a cooking pot and add vegetable broth so that carrots are completely immersed.

Cover and bring to a boil, then simmer at low heat for approximately 45 minutes. Once carrots are cooked, mix the whole thing in a blender; look to create a creamy-like consistency.

Immediately before serving, add just enough coconut milk to give it a light coconut taste. Stir so that both coconut milk and carrot preparation are well mixed. Add *freshly ground black pepper* and *sea salt* to taste.

A variant: no coconut, no pepper, but add freshly crushed caraway instead (at the beginning, with carrots and broth, add approx. 2 teaspoons of caraway for every 2 lbs of carrots).

Leek & Potato Soup

- *2 leeks*
- *2-3 medium-sized white potatoes*
- *16 oz. (474 ml) of vegetable broth*
- *1-2 bay leaves*
- *1 clove of garlic*
- *Dry chives*

In a cooking pot, sauté finely chopped leeks at high intensity in *butter* until brown. Stir regularly so nothing sticks and burns. Then, reduce heat to medium and sweat leeks. When almost done, add crushed garlic (not before, because garlic burns easily).

Add vegetable broth, coarsely chopped potatoes, bay leaves, 2−3 tablespoons of dry chives, and finish by adding water (approximately half the amount used for vegetable broth). Cover and bring to a boil.

Next, reduce heat and simmer until potatoes are cooked.

When ready, remove bay leaves and mix soup in a blender. Add *sea salt* and *freshly ground pepper* to taste. Adjust consistency by adding more vegetable broth or water.

Just before serving, decorate each soup with dry chives.

Lentil Soup

Rinse 2 cups of uncooked **lentils** (of your choice) in a strainer and remove all inedible debris (like rocks or wrinkled lentils). No need for soaking.

Prepare veggies by finely chopping:

- *2 big French shallots* (when chopping, do not mix with other vegetables)
- *3 celery sticks* (include leaves)
- *2 sweet colored bell peppers*
- *2-3 big carrots*

In a cooking pot, gently sauté French shallots and crushed garlic at high intensity in **vegetable oil** (of your choice) until brown. Stir regularly so that nothing will stick and burn. Add all veggies and keep on stirring at high intensity for a few minutes, until they become somewhat brownish on the outside, but also remain crispy; avoid cooking too long and having the veggies become soft.

Next, add *50 oz. (1.5 L) of vegetable broth*, *17 oz. (0.5 L) of water*, *2 bay leaves*, a big bouquet of *fresh thyme* and any combination of the following dried herbs: *sweet marjoram*, *parsley*, *oregano*, *rosemary*. Add lentils also.

Cover and bring to a boil, then simmer for 30-60 minutes (depending on your preferred consistency of lentils; I use green lentils and I like them after about 50 minutes). Adjust soup consistency with vegetable broth or water (I often end up adding at least 1 cup). Add *sea salt* and *fleshly ground black pepper* to taste. Remove bay leaves and thyme stems before serving.

Hot Soups

Wild Mushroom Soup with Rosemary

- *1.4 oz. (40 g) dried wild mushrooms* (boletus, forest mix)
- *24 oz. (680 g) fresh mushrooms of your choice*
- *Freshly squeezed lemon juice*
- *Vegetable broth*
- *2–3 medium-sized potatoes*
- *Dried rosemary*
- *Butter*
- *Sea salt & freshly ground black pepper*

Pan-fry or sauté (in butter) a generous amount of fresh mushrooms of your choice (not the dried wild mushrooms). I use the term "generous" here because mushrooms, through cooking, reduce to approximately a third of their initial size. Once ready, deglaze at high temperature with freshly squeezed lemon juice (approx. 1 lemon wedge).

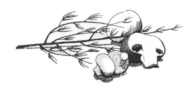

Next, in a cooking pot, mix sautéed mushrooms, dried wild mushrooms and coarsely chopped potatoes. Then, add vegetable broth to desired consistency. The potatoes will serve to thicken the soup. Add enough dried rosemary to create a nice balance of taste and aromas... not too much to overshadow mushrooms. Cook at low temperature for a minimum of 1 hour.

Then, mix the whole thing in a blender. Adjust to taste with sea salt, freshly ground pepper, freshly squeezed lemon juice, butter and dried rosemary.

Yellow Beet Soup

Put cubes of **peeled raw yellow beets** in a cooking pot. Add enough **vegetable broth** to completely immerse beets. Cover and bring to a boil. Next, reduce heat and simmer for 1 hour. Finally, purée in blender, and it's ready to serve!

Recipes: Appetizers, Snacks and Side Dishes

Alfalfa & Avocado Spread

Create this spread by mixing **guacamole** (see Guacamole recipe in this section, but leave the coriander and red bell pepper out for this preparation) and **alfalfa sprouts** together.

Use either as sandwich spread, on **crackers** as canapés, or inside a rolled-up **romaine lettuce leaf** as cigar-shaped finger food. You may also use to stuff baked **baby potatoes**, adding **freshly ground black pepper**.

Approximate gastric evacuation time: 4 hours.

Asparagus & Pine Nuts with Truffle Oil

Steam small **asparagus spears** (choose firm spears with closed, compact tips; you may also use **green beans** instead of asparagus) until *al dente*.

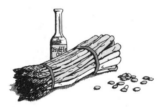

Serve in a plate; sprinkle with **black truffle oil**, **fresh pine nuts** (roasted lightly in the oven on a cookie sheet, or using stove in a dry pan, just prior to making recipe) or **freshly crushed almonds**, **sea salt** and **freshly ground black pepper**.

Approximate gastric evacuation time: 4 ½ hours. Although proteins are listed as 6 hours, nuts usually leave the stomach quicker than other proteins, such as animal products, especially if eaten with high-water content vegetables like asparagus.

Braised Fennel with Orange & Almonds

Lay large pieces of **fennel bulbs** in a cooking dish.

Sprinkle with:

- *Orange juice* (freshly squeezed or other, your choice)
- *Lemon* & *orange zests*
- *Sea salt*
- *Olive oil*

Cook at 375 °F. Baste occasionally (with cooking juices). Fennel will be ready when soft enough to pierce with a fork. Sprinkle with freshly crushed or finely sliced **almonds** and then broil until almonds become light brown. Adjust by seasoning with **sea salt** and **freshly ground black pepper**.

Approximate gastric evacuation time: 4 ½ hours.

Buffalo Mozzarella & Tomato

Buffalo mozzarella is an Italian mozzarella cheese made from buffalo milk. This is a delicacy for cheese amateurs. It is common, however, to find very bland versions of this cheese, so look only for high quality and select carefully; sample in-store if possible.

In a plate, prepare a bed of **baby arugula.** Lay cheese slices (for tastier results, it is very important that cheese be at room temperature), alternating with **red tomato** slices. Add **olive oil**, a hint of **balsamic vinegar**, **sea salt** and **freshly ground black pepper**.

Cheese Made from Raw Milk

I find cheese made from raw milk to be tastier than pasteurized cheese. For weight loss purposes, the former is better, as heating (pasteurization) tends to destroy nutrients and clump proteins together (making for more difficult digestion).

Cheese Plate

This is for you cheese lovers (as I am!). Please note that there is a whole world of cheese to be discovered beyond mozzarella, cheddar, Havarti and Monterey Jack... There are many different groups of cheese and, within these groups, various types according to their milk origin, fabrication, maturing process, etc.

Cheeses are usually made from the milk of cows, buffalos, goats, and/or sheep. The nomenclature and classifications for cheese groups may vary from one country to the next. Because there are so many different varieties, I will not list them here. Instead, I suggest you go down to your local cheese store and discover for yourself...some stores carry over 200 different types!

Serving recommendations:

- Cheese is better served at "room temperature," or around 50 °F−60 °F (10 °C−15 °C). Avoid serving "right out of the refrigerator" (colder temperature makes cheese less flavorful) or too warm (higher temperature makes it "sweat" and lose valuable water).

- Because cheese is a low-water content food, balance out by serving with **high-water content vegetables**, like tomatoes, celery and cucumber. Cheese (protein) and bread (starchy food) are NOT to be eaten together, of course.

Approximate gastric evacuation time: 5 hours. Animal products, like meats and eggs, have an approximate time of 6 hours. Cheese, being a little easier to digest however, goes through more rapidly (unless you are lactose intolerant), especially if eaten with high-water content vegetables.

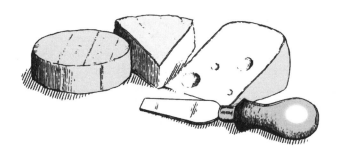

Eggplant & Tomato Canapé

Cut *eggplant* into thin slices. Then, either sauté in a large skillet with *vegetable oil*, or cook in oven at 425 °F on a cookie sheet (also with *vegetable oil*).

Once cooked, add *sea salt* and *freshly squeezed lemon juice* to taste.

On bite-sized *crackers* (e.g., www.ryvita.com), spread a little *butter*, *avocado* or *olive oil spread* (e.g., www.solidolive.com), and add a slice of cooked eggplant. Top off with a piece of *sweet tomato*. Season with *sea salt* and *freshly ground black pepper*.

Approximate gastric evacuation time: 5 hours. Crackers and fats (butter, avocado) are listed at 4 hours, but the presence of many fats, along with the acid/starchy combination of tomatoes/crackers, prolongs this duration.

Focaccia

Focaccia is a flat oven baked Italian bread.

Spread *olive oil* to cover selected amount of *pita breads*, and sprinkle with a mix of *crushed sea salt* and *dried rosemary*.

Place in oven at 200 °F for a few minutes, just enough so they get warm and crispy. Make sure to keep an eye on them as pitas burn easily.

Cut pitas in pie-slice-shaped pieces and serve. They are great with pasta, salads and dips.

Approximate gastric evacuation time: 4 hours.

Grilled Vegetable Antipasto

In Italy, the first course of a meal is called "antipasto". It is generally composed of marinated vegetables, olives, various cheeses, cured meats and bruschetta. We will create our own here by serving grilled vegetables with oil.

In a bowl, mix:

Thin long pieces of **colored carrots** (orange, yellow, purple, etc.) and **colored sweet bell peppers**

Slices of **onions** and **mushrooms**

Medium-sized **asparagus spears**

Thick long pieces of e**ggplant** and **zucchini**

Then add the following seasoning:

- *Sea salt*
- *Freshly ground black pepper*
- *Fresh garlic*
- *Fresh basil, oregano and rosemary*
- *Olive oil*

Mix well and spread evenly on a large cooking sheet. Place in oven at 375 °F for 30 minutes.

Remove from oven. Directly on cooking sheet and with a spatula, move vegetables around a little. If they tend to stick, add vegetable oil. Spread evenly again on cooking sheet and stick in oven for another 15 minutes.

Remove once more from oven. Mix again, same as before. By this time, they should have a wilted look. Spread evenly and cook one last time for 10−15 minutes. To get a grilled look, broiling may be needed for a few minutes before removing from oven.

Add a few drops of **freshly squeezed lemon juice**, and serve.

You may serve them in individual-sized bowls, on pasta or as a salad on a bed of lettuce. You may also accompany them with focaccia, crackers or pieces of bread (lightly toasted).

Approximate gastric evacuation time: 3 hours.
With pasta, bread or crackers: 4 hours.

Guacamole

Guacamole is an avocado-based Mexican dip.

In a bowl, mix:

- *Mashed soft ripe avocados*
- *Freshly squeezed lemon or lime juice*
- *Sea salt*
- *Freshly ground coriander seeds*
- *Fine-cut red bell peppers* (optional)

Spread on **Focaccia**, **crackers** or **lightly toasted bread pieces**, or eat as a vegetable dip with **sweet bell pepper**, **carrots**, **cucumber** and **celery sticks**.

Approximate gastric evacuation time: 4 hours.
With bread or crackers: 5 hours.

Vegetable Juices

For these recipes, get your hands on a juice extractor and create a host of various juices. For example:

- *Carrots* by themselves
- *Sweet bell peppers* with *carrots* and *celery*
- *Sweet bell peppers* with *cucumber* and *celery*
- *Yellow beets* by themselves
- *Etc.*

Approximate gastric evacuation time: 1½ hours. Non-starchy vegetables are listed at 3 hours; in their liquid form, however, they evacuate more rapidly from the stomach.

Recipes: Salads

For many, the word "salad" evokes images of something bland and monotonous. If you fall into this category, we invite you to scroll through this section and see if you can't re-invent the salad as something original and delicious. One of the tricks, for example, is to steer off the path of common salad items (like iceberg lettuce, vinegar based dressings and bland tomatoes), as these are either weight promoting or flavorless; as you will see, *fewer tastier* ingredients is the way to go.

On the other hand, you may already be a salad lover but, after having read Step 3, realized that most of the salads you have ever eaten were fattening, and now you're wondering what type of salad you can eat in order to lose weight. Fear not, for we have a few options for you. Salads with only veggies have an approximate gastric evacuation time of 3 hours. Add any low-water content foods (like bread, potatoes, nuts or cheese), and you may count 4 hours. Although items like nuts, cheese and cream usually have a longer gastric evacuation period, this time is decreased when eaten with high-water content vegetables (such as lettuce, cucumber and celery). Because of their fruit content, do not eat any other type of food with either the Citrus & Avocado Salad or the Mango Salad.

Barley & Carrot Salad

The most popular form of barley in America is pearl barley. It takes 30–45 minutes to cook (two parts of water for one part of uncooked barley). Cool down on counter top until heat vapors dissipate and set in refrigerator to chill.

In a salad bowl, mix the following:

- *2 cups of chilled cooked barley*
- *Olive oil*
- *Finely chopped fresh Italian parsley and basil*
- *Freshly squeezed lemon juice* (1–2 wedges)
- *Sea salt*
- *Freshly ground black pepper*

Caesar Salad

Create a Caesar-like dressing by mixing the following ingredients:

- *Finely grated Parmesan cheese*
- *Olive oil*
- *A hint of Dijon mustard*
- *Freshly ground black pepper*
- *Freshly crushed garlic*
- *Sea salt*
- *Freshly squeezed lemon juice*

Mix in generously with **romaine lettuce**, and sprinkle any remaining grated Parmesan cheese.

Cherry Tomato & Parmesan Salad

In a salad bowl, mix **red cherry tomatoes** with **roughly cut pieces of Parmesan cheese**, **fresh basil**, **olive oil** and **sea salt**. Simple and delicious!

Citrus & Avocado Salad

In a salad bowl, mix:

- *Lettuce*
- *Chopped cucumberDices of soft ripe avocado*
- *Pieces of citrus* (any combination of clementine, orange, pink grapefruit, mandarine and tangerine)

Add s*ea salt* and *freshly ground black pepper* to taste.

Creamy Cucumber Salad with Dill

This is a simple and refreshing salad made of mainly cucumber and lettuce.

Create a dressing with the following:

- *Olive oil*
- *Sea salt*
- *Freshly ground black pepper*
- *35% cream*
- *Freshly squeezed lemon juice*
- *Fresh or dry dill*

Garden Salad

In a salad bowl, mix any of the following fresh vegetables. You may mix them all but, if you want to keep salad down to a reasonable size and have less cutting to do, choose 5–6.

- *Alfalfa sprouts*
- *Green bean*
- *Avocado*
- *Lettuce* (of your choice)
- *Bean sprouts*
- *Mushrooms*
- *Broccoli*

- *Sweet bell pepper*
- *Carrot*
- *Sweet peas* (in the pod)
- *Cauliflower*
- *Sweet tomato*
- *Celery*
- *Yellow beet*
- *Cucumber*

Create salad dressing with **vegetable oil**, **sea salt** and **freshly squeezed lemon juice.** You may also use **fresh herbs** like basil, thyme, oregano, rosemary, cilantro, and even a hint of **maple syrup**.

This salad can be served with **crackers**, **bread** (lightly toasted) or **focaccia** (as described in the Appetizers, Snacks & Side Dishes section).

Lentil Salad with Fine Herbs

Soak and cook **lentils** (of your choice) according to package instructions.

Then, make the following infusion of fresh herbs: in a small cooking pot, warm **vegetable oil** at low heat. Remove from heat and add **fresh herbs** (e.g., oregano, thyme, sweet marjoram, and rosemary). Be careful not to overheat, as fresh herbs burn easily. "Warm" is warm enough to stick your finger in the oil without burning it, no more.

Next, mix herbal infusion with cooked lentils and add diced **celery**, **cucumber** and **sweet bell peppers**. Complete with **freshly squeezed lemon juice**, **sea salt** and **freshly ground pepper**.

Serve as a lukewarm salad (hot lentils + cold veggies = lukewarm) or as a chilled refreshing salad (pre-cooked just out-of-the-fridge lentils and herbs, with cold veggies).

In this salad, you may also substitute lentils for grains, like **barley** or **quinoa**.

Mango Dressing Salad

Create this delicious mango dressing by mixing the following ingredients in a blender:

- *Mango* (use less fibrous variety, like Haden or Atulfo)
- *Fresh sage or basil*
- *Sea salt*
- *Freshly ground black pepper*

In a salad bowl, mix **lettuce**, chopped **celery**, **cucumber** and diced **soft ripe avocado**. Add mango dressing.

Market Salad

In a salad bowl, mix <u>any</u> of the following fresh vegetables:

- *Alfalfa sprouts*
- *Snow peas*
- *Bean sprouts*
- *Heart of palm*
- *Broccoli*
- *Lettuce* (of your choice)
- *Cauliflower*
- *Mushrooms*
- *Celery*
- *Tomato* (of your choice)
- *Cucumber*
- *Sweet bell pepper*

Salad dressing: **vegetable oil**, **sea salt** and **freshly squeezed lemon juice**. You may also add a hint of **Dijon mustard**, **unsweetened soy sauce** and/or **sun-dried tomatoes**.

Turn this salad into a protein meal by adding either **fresh nuts** (of your choice, but no peanuts) or **cheese pieces** (see Cheese Plate recipe for tips on cheese selection).

Potato Salad

Steam 1–2 lbs of **baby potatoes** (white or red, with skin). When ready, cut into halves.

In a skillet, sauté thin slices of **leek** (at least 2 medium-sized) and **mushrooms** (2 generous handfuls of button, Portobello or oyster mushrooms) in **vegetable oil**. When almost ready, add the potatoes to brown them a little. Deglaze with **lemon juice** or **balsamic vinegar**.

Add **garlic salt** generously and finish with **sea salt** and **freshly ground black pepper** to taste.

In a salad bowl, prepare a bed of **lettuce** (of your choice) and cover with the potato and leek sauté. Adjust with additional vegetable oil and garlic salt.

Tabbouleh

Commonly, tabbouleh is a salad of fine-ground bulgur (cracked wheat grains), parsley, tomatoes, green onions, mint, olive oil, and lemon juice.

Cook **bulgur** or **couscous** in **vegetable broth** as indicated on package. Set in refrigerator to chill.

Once chilled, in a large salad bowl, mix the following ingredients with bulgur:

- *Sweet tomatoes*
- *Diced peeled cucumber*
- *Minced fresh Italian parsley*
- *A hint of fresh mint*
- *Sea salt*
- *Vegetable oil*
- *Freshly squeezed lemon juice*
- *Lemon zest*

Walnut & Celery Salad with Cheese

In a salad bowl, mix 1 part of each of the following: *finely chopped celery*, *walnut pieces* and *grated Gruyere cheese*.

Make dressing with:

- *2 parts olive oil*
- *1 part Dijon mustard*
- *Freshly squeezed lemon juice* (1–2 wedges)
- *Sea salt*
- *Freshly ground black pepper*

Warm Eggplant Salad

In a skillet, sauté *diced eggplant* in *vegetable oil*.

In a salad bowl, mix sautéed eggplant with:

- *A generous amount of alfalfa sprouts*
- *1 diced sweet bell pepper*
- *1–2 diced sweet tomatoes*
- *Fresh basil and/or oregano*

Create salad dressing with *olive oil*, *freshly squeezed lemon juice* and *sea salt*.

Transform this salad into a pasta meal by replacing the tomato and alfalfa sprouts with cooked pasta of your choice.

Warm Mushroom Salad

In a pan, sauté sliced *mushrooms* of your choice (button, portobello, oyster, etc.) in *vegetable oil*.

In a salad bowl, prepare a generous bed of *lettuce* and add diced *soft ripe avocado*. Cover with sautéed mushrooms.

Make salad dressing with *grilled sesame oil*, *freshly squeezed limejuice* and *sea salt*.

Recipes: Sandwiches

For sandwiches in this section, allow approximately 6 hours of gastric evacuation time. Bread is listed in Step 3 as having a gastric evacuation time of approximately 4 hours, but most of the following sandwiches have other ingredients that slow this process. Vegenaise, tomatoes or lemon juice (acids with starchy food are not ideal but acceptable for weight loss in these recipes).

BLT

- *Lightly toasted bread* (very good with spelt bread)
- *Lettuce*
- *Vegenaise* (www.followyourheart.com)
- *Tomato slices*
- *Grilled & smoked coconuts bits* (replaces bacon, sold in some food stores; another option is *Bac'Uns* at www.frontiercoop.com)
- *Sea salt & freshly ground black pepper*

Spread Vegenaise generously over each bread slice. Cover one bread slice with ¼ inch of smoked coconut (compact neatly so it doesn't fall off). Add lettuce and tomato slices, salt and pepper, and top with second bread slice.

Chips

Chips and sandwiches are a popular duo. For weight loss purposes, I do not recommend you eat chips often, but occasionally is OK. Stay away from anything too radical, like spicy Thai, hot anything, salt & vinegar, cheddar, etc.; instead, choose regular (plain, nothing added), sea salt or with herbs. Here are some brands I particularly like:

Solea: www.goodhealthnaturalproducts.com
Kettle: www.kettlefoods.com

Club Sandwich

For this modified version of the common recipe, you'll need:

- *3 bread slices, lightly toasted* (good with spelt bread)
- *Tomato slices*
- *Lettuce*
- *Vegenaise* (www.followyourheart.com)
- *Grilled & smoked coconuts bits* (replaces bacon, sold in some food stores; another option is *Bac'Uns* at www.frontiercoop.com)
- *Sea salt & freshly ground black pepper* And as a substitute for chicken: *grilled eggplant slices*, cooked in *vegetable oil* at medium-high in a large skillet (or in the oven at 450 °F).

Spread Vegenaise generously over 1 side of each toasted bread slice. Cover first bread slice with ¼ inch of smoked coconut (compact neatly so it doesn't fall off). Top with stack of lettuce, then add tomato slices, and season with salt and pepper.

Place second toasted bread slice and cover with eggplant. Add salt and pepper. Finish by layering with lettuce and covering with third toasted bread slice (Vegenaise facing downward, of course).

Pin sandwich's layers together by piercing with 4 frill picks.

Grilled Vegetable Sandwich

To create enough garnishing for 2 sandwiches, you'll need:

- *1 sweet onion*
- *4 handfuls of uncooked mushrooms*

(I find oyster mushrooms or button mushrooms to be particularly good for this recipe)

- *1 sweet bell pepper*
- *Freshly squeezed lemon juice*
- *Fresh herbs, like oregano, thyme & rosemary*
- *Sea salt*
- *Freshly ground black pepper*

In a large skillet, sauté thin slices of sweet onions in **vegetable oil** until they become brown, but not quite a burned color. Add mushroom slices (remember that mushrooms will reduce to a third when cooked, so plan your quantities accordingly).

A few minutes before mushrooms are done, add strips of sweet bell pepper and cook *al dente*.

Deglaze with freshly squeezed lemon juice (approx. 1 lemon wedge) and add fresh herbs. Season with sea salt and freshly ground black pepper.

On lightly toasted **bread**, spread **olive oil** and garnish with the onion/mushroom/sweet bell pepper mix.

Mediterranean Open Face Sandwich

Be creative by adding any other grilled veggies like **eggplant** and **zucchini.**

Toast **bread** slices lightly and spread **mashed soft ripe avocado** on each.

Add the following to each toasted bread slice:

- *Sweet tomato slices* (yellow or orange)
- *Fresh basil* (wholes leaves)
- *Sea salt*
- *Freshly ground black pepper*
- *Olive oil*
- *A few drops of freshly squeezed lemon juice*

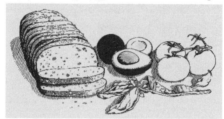

Mushroom Burger

In this recipe, **portobello mushrooms** will serve as the burger patty. Because mushrooms reduce while cooking, choose bigger ones. Begin by removing stems from mushrooms. You may then leave mushrooms whole or cut them in thick slices (which reduces cooking time).

Mix the following ingredients in a bowl (establish quantities according to the number of burgers to be eaten).

- *Vegetable oil*
- *Fresh thyme*
- *Crushed garlic*
- *Sea salt*

- *Freshly ground black pepper*

Brush insides of **burger buns** and entire surface of Portobello mushrooms with this mix. Select healthy burger buns (the fewer ingredients, the better). Look for no more ingredients than: integral flour, water, yeast and sea salt.

Then, prepare **slices of sweet tomatoes,** fresh **lettuce leaves** and chopped **sun-dried tomatoes**. Set aside as these will be added later to burger assembly.

In a large skillet, sauté thin slices of **sweet onions** in **vegetable oil** until brown, but not quite a burned color. Deglaze with **freshly squeezed lemon juice** (approx. 1 lemon wedge), add **sea salt**, and then set aside.

Next, sauté portobello mushrooms (optional: instead of being only brushed, mushrooms may also be marinated a day—or at least a few hours—before cooking).

Before assembling burger, lightly toast burger buns (with thyme and garlic preparation) in oven; then spread **Vegenaise** on both pieces.

The assembly should have layers as follows:

Top Burger Bun
Vegenaise
Salt & Pepper
Sun-Dried Tomatoes
Onions
Tomato Slices
Portobello Mushrooms
Lettuce Leaves
Vegenaise
Bottom Burger Bun

And enjoy!

177

Recipes: Varied Dishes

Allow 5 hours of gastric evacuation time for all recipes in this section. Although starchy foods are listed as 4 hours, this time is extended due to the presence of other ingredients, like butter and cream; corn-on-the-cob remains 4 hours because of its higher water content. Cheese and tofu, although listed with other proteins as 6 hours, leave the stomach a little bit faster, which accounts for the 5 hours we recommend here.

Brussels Sprouts & Mushrooms au Gratin

Steam **Brussels sprouts** until *al dente*, and then cut into halves.

In a salad bowl, mix Brussels sprouts with:

- *Finely chopped button mushrooms*
- *Finely chopped fresh Italian parsley*
- *Melted butter*
- *A hint of Dijon mustard*
- *Sea salt*

Transfer to a cooking plate and cover with grated **Gruyere cheese** (preferably made from raw milk), and sprinkle **freshly ground black pepper**. Stick in oven at 350 °F until cheese is melted, then broil so corners turn to light brown.

Corn-on-the-Cob

Very simple here...steamed **fresh corn-on-the-cob** with **butter** and a little **sea salt**. A delicious treat and great for weight loss!

Garden Couscous

Couscous is available in most food stores.

Cook **couscous** in **vegetable broth** according to package instructions.

Steam **asparagus spears** until *al dente*, and then cut into small pieces.

Sauté sliced **mushrooms** in a skillet with **butter**. Just before they are done, add small pieces of **colored bell pepper**; sauté these only a few seconds (not too long, so they remain crisp).

On a big serving plate, mix couscous and vegetables; add **butter**, **sea salt**, **freshly ground black pepper** and serve.

Oriental Tofu

Cut **regular firm** or **extra firm tofu** into bite-sized pieces and store in an airtight container (e.g., Tupperware®).

Create marinade (enough to completely cover tofu) with:

- *1 part toasted sesame oil*
- *1 part freshly squeezed lemon and/or lime juice*
- *1 part unsweetened soy sauce*
- *Lemon and/or lime zests*
- *Freshly ground coriander seeds, to taste*

...cover tofu and let marinate for a minimum of 24 hours in refrigerator.

24 hours later, in a big cooking wok, sweat a few **onions** in **vegetable oil**, add **sliced mushrooms** and sauté.

Next, mix in and stir-fry marinated tofu; deglaze with marinade.

When almost done, add a few thin slices of **yellow bell peppers** and a generous portion of sliced **bok choy** (Chinese cabbage). For a final touch, add **beans sprouts**.

Adjust seasoning with any of the marinade ingredients, and **sea salt** to taste.

Pizza

This recipe makes four medium-sized pizzas.

For pizza crust, use thin medium-sized (approx. 9 inch) of either of the following: **homemade pizza dough**, **ready-made pizza crust** (from a Health food store) or **large pita bread**. Either way, make sure these are made with as little ingredients as possible (e.g., flour, salt, yeast, oil, and water). No dairy products or eggs. If you make your own, you must pre-cook in order to make this recipe.

For pizza sauce, you will need:

- *4 red bell peppers*
- *2 sliced leeks*
- *4 freshly crushed garlic cloves*
- *Sea salt*
- *Freshly ground pepper*

Cut bell peppers into halves (lengthwise), remove seeds and stems, and place on a large cooking sheet (facing down). Set oven grill at top level. Broil until skin gets evenly dark brown and is burned (without setting fire to your kitchen...) so the skin will easily come off; keep an eye on the rest of the bell peppers so they do not burn. Take out from the oven, cool down, remove and throw away skin.

While bell peppers are cooling down, sauté leeks in skillet with freshly crushed garlic cloves. When leeks are tenderly cooked, add sea salt, and remove from heat.

In a blender, mix cooked bell peppers with leek preparation. Add sea salt and freshly ground pepper to taste.

This pizza sauce may also serve as a pasta sauce or simply as soup with croutons. Therefore, if you like it, make a bigger batch.

For pizza toppings, slice **10 portobello mushrooms** and **5 regular-sized onions** (you may also vary by swapping mushrooms for zucchini or eggplant). Separate onion rings. Mix in salad bowl with *vegetable oil* and sea salt. Spread on cooking sheet. Place in oven at 425 °F. Turn over slices so as to cook on both sides, until tender and a bit crispy on the outside.

To assemble pizza, cover pizza crust generously with pizza sauce, spread grilled onions and mushrooms evenly, and pour **35% cream** in a trickle fashion to cover the entire surface. Add sea salt, freshly ground pepper, **garlic salt** and coarsely chopped **fresh basil leaves**. Place in oven at 400 °F for 7−12 minutes, or until crust is crispy. Just before serving, add a trickle of **black truffle oil**...yummy delicious!

Suggested accompaniment: a refreshing salad made of **lettuce**, **cucumber**, **olive oil**, **35% cream**, **freshly squeezed lemon or lime juice**, **sea salt** and **freshly ground pepper**.

Potato Purée with Truffle Oil

Steam bite-sized pieces of **Yukon Gold potatoes** (with skin) and 1−2 **garlic cloves** (also with skin...even the most outer thin paper-like layer). Yukon Golds are also called Yellow Finnish potatoes; they have a naturally buttery flavor and moist texture that makes them excellent for mashing.

Once potatoes and garlic are cooked, peel garlic and mix both, adding:

- *Olive oil or butter* (add to desired consistency)
- *Black truffle oil* (add to desired flavor; use sparingly)
- *Sea salt*
- *Freshly ground black pepper*

...and then mash.

Suggestion: serve with a Garden Salad (see Salads section).

Rice & Wild Mushrooms

Cook **rice** (I especially like short-grain brown rice) in **vegetable broth**, with **dried mushrooms** and 3–4 knobs of **butter**. When using rice in various recipes, look also for assorted rice grain packages; older rice varieties with different shapes, colors and taste...know there is a whole realm beyond regular white rice!

While rice is cooking, sauté sliced **mushrooms** (button, portobello, oyster, boletus, etc.) in a large skillet. Because of cooking shrinkage, use plenty. Once mushrooms are done, deglaze with **freshly squeezed lemon juice** (approx. 2 lemon wedges) and add **sea salt**.

Next, add cooked rice to mushrooms in the skillet, and mix. Adjust with butter, freshly squeezed lemon juice and sea salt.

A variant: brown basmati rice with sautéed mushrooms, vegetable oil or butter, fresh thyme and sea salt.

Sautéed Potatoes with Thyme

Cut **potatoes** into small cubes (leave skin), and place in cooking pan. Add minced green onions. Sprinkle **vegetable oil** or pieces of **butter** (the butter will blend in well as you stir potatoes and turn them over during cooking); add **fresh thyme** and **sea salt**.

Cook in oven at 400 °F—450 °F.

With a spatula, turn potatoes over occasionally to cook evenly on all sides, and to prevent them from sticking to the pan.

Shepherd's Pie

Steam **Yukon Gold** or **White potatoes**. Mix with **butter** or **vegetable oil** and **sea salt**, and mash. Look to create a creamy result. As an option, add a few drops of **black truffle oil**.

In a large skillet, sauté a few **onions** in vegetable oil at medium-high heat until brown. Add sliced **button mushrooms**, and keep on sautéing. Once the mushrooms are ready, deglaze with *freshly squeezed lemon juice* (approx. 1 lemon wedge). *Salt* lightly.

Next, assemble Shepherd's pie:

Bottom layer – Lay the mushroom/onion mix at the bottom of a large baking dish. With a flat spatula, make sure this layer is neatly compacted.

Middle layer – Add *corn* (regular canned corn will do; use a brand that has nothing but corn - water and salt is OK, but no sugar). Again, make sure this layer is neatly compacted.

Top layer – Add potato mix. Compact once more. Sprinkle *freshly grounded pepper*.

Stick in oven at 350 °F for approximately 15 minutes and, just before removing, broil for a few minutes so potatoes turn to light brown.

Recipes: Pasta

All dishes in this section have a gastric evacuation time of approximately 5 hours. Pasta by itself has an approximate time of 4 hours but, given that these recipes are made up of many other ingredients (i.e., concentrated foods like vegetable oils and cream and irritants like garlic and pepper), we suggest you extend this to 5 hours.

Angel Hair Primavera

Cook **angel hair pasta** until *al dente*.

In a large skillet, stir-fry small pieces of **broccoli** with **freshly crushed garlic** in **butter** or **olive oil** at medium-high temperature.

Cut very thin strips of **yellow** and/or **green zucchini** and **carrots**; add to broccoli, and stir-fry. Add a few strips of **colored bell peppers** and stir-fry just enough so they become warm but stay crisp. Deglaze with **freshly squeezed lemon juice** (approx. 2 lemon wedges).

In a skillet, mix pasta with vegetables at low heat. Add 1−2 teaspoon of **grated lemon peel**, butter or olive oil (use same as used with vegetable stir-fry), **sea salt**, **fresh oregano, fresh basil** and **freshly ground black pepper**.

Fettuccine with Creamy Avocado Sauce

In a blender, purée:

- **Soft ripe avocados**
- **Red bell pepper**
- **Sweet grape tomatoes** (or any other low acid tomato)
- **Freshly squeezed lemon juice**
- **Sea salt**
- **Vegetable oil**

Add just enough vegetables to create a creamy texture...not too watery. As a variant, you may also add cucumber and/or celery.

Cook **fettuccine pasta** until *al dente*. Then, put pasta in serving plates, cover with avocado sauce and top off with a little **fresh basil** and a few finely chopped **sun-dried tomatoes**.

Fusilli & Bell Pepper Salad

Cook *fusilli pasta* (swirl shaped) until *al dente*. Rinse under cold water to stop cooking process, and to cool them off.

In a large salad bowl, mix pasta with:

- *Finely cut colored bell peppers*
- *Vegetable oil*
- *Freshly squeezed lemon juice*
- *Freshly crushed coriander seeds*
- *Sea salt*
- *A hint of maple syrup* (or brown sugar)

Linguine with Creamy Sauce

Cook **linguini pasta** until *al dente*.

To create sauce, sauté in a large skillet **2 finely sliced leeks** in **vegetable oil**. When tender, add 4 oz. (118 ml) of **35% cream** and **2 mashed ripe avocados**. Stir enough so that texture is smooth and homogenized.

Season with:

- *Freshly ground coriander seeds*
- *Lemongrass*
- *Sea salt*
- *Freshly ground black pepper*
- *Garlic salt*

...and finally, just before pouring on pasta, add **2 other ripe avocados** cut into small cubes.

Pasta with Rosée Sauce

To make enough rosée sauce for 2 people, you will need:

- *6 finely chopped French shallots*
- *3 crushed garlic cloves*
- *16 oz. (473 ml) of 35% cream*
- *Dried oregano and fresh basil*
- *Freshly ground black pepper* and *sea salt*
- *2 handfuls of small red tomatoes* (grape variety is best)
- *1 handful of sun-dried tomatoes*

Begin by sautéing French shallots and garlic in a large skillet at medium-high temperature in **butter**. Keep stirring so garlic doesn't stick and burn. When onions are tender, pour cream in slowly, and add dried oregano, freshly ground pepper and sea salt. Adjust heat and make a reduction for 10−15 minutes while stirring regularly so that cream doesn't stick.

Cook pasta of your choosing, al dente.

To the side, purée both fresh and sun-dried tomatoes in blender, along with fresh basil.

Remove skillet from heat and pour tomato purée slowly into cream preparation while stirring, until you reach an even, light pink color.

Set the cooked pasta in a pasta bowl and cover generously with sauce.

Pasta

Recipes: For Carnivores

When it comes to animal products, I recommend buying organic, grain-fed and/or free-range, as these have less chances of having hormone or pesticide residues. Also, try diet-style cooking: avoid frying, breading or using oil/cream-based sauces; instead, use steaming, grilling or aluminum foil techniques. You may use fresh herbs, lemon juice, and light spices and mustard to bake "en croûte" (a thin crust will form as cooking occurs).

Animal products are full of hard-to-digest substances (i.e., cholesterol, saturated fats, colorants & dyes, preservatives, hormone & pesticide residues, etc.), and these make for a long gastric evacuation time. In addition, proteins exposed to heat (as in cooking) tend to coagulate and form a dense mass, making meat, seafood, fish and poultry even harder to digest. In order for the recipes in this section to have their weight loss effect, factor in a good 7 hours of gastric evacuation time. If eaten alone, these food items are listed at 6 hours, but given that there are other ingredients in the recipes, add the extra hour.

Buttered Tilapia with Curry

On a large piece of aluminum foil, create a bed of **sliced green onions** and lay **fresh Tilapia fillets** (or any other white-fleshed fish). Sprinkle with **yellow curry powder** and **sea salt**, and add knobs (see Cooking Glossary) of **butter** on each fillet. Fold the aluminum over so as to leave no opening.

Place in oven at 375 °F for approximately 20 minutes. Fish is cooked when flesh is no longer translucent, but opaque.

Serve by adding more sea salt and butter (if needed), along with steamed **asparagus**, **green beans** or **Brussels sprouts**, also with butter.

Pepper Steak & Mushrooms

In a skillet, over medium-high heat, cook **finely sliced French shallots** (until tender) and **mushrooms** (button or portobello) in **butter**. When done, empty skillet contents in a bowl (don't rinse skillet just yet).

Sprinkle **rib-eye steak** generously with **freshly ground pepper**, a few **lemon zests** and a little bit of **sea salt**. In the same skillet, over medium-high heat (still in butter), cook steak until browned on both sides, and according to personal preference (rare, medium, well-done, or anywhere in between). Place steak on warmed platter and cover to keep warm.

Reduce heat to medium. Deglaze with **balsamic vinegar**. Cook 1 minute, stirring to loosen brown bits on bottom of skillet. To thicken, add a knob of butter.

In a serving plate, spread French shallot and mushroom mixture over steak, and then cover with cooking reduction.

This preparation, of course, may also be used for any other beef or wild game (e.g., venison, bison and deer) cuts.

Poultry Marinated with Dijon & Herbs

You may use any **poultry of your preference**, including chicken, duck, turkey, pheasant, quail, partridge, etc.

Create marinade with:

- *Dijon mustard*
- *Freshly crushed juniper berries*
- *Fresh thyme*
- *Fresh rosemary*
- *Bay leaves*
- *Sea salt*
- *Freshly ground black pepper*

Be generous with all ingredients (except for salt because mustard is already somewhat salty).

Cut poultry into cubes of about 1 inch by 1 inch. Cover with marinade, and set in refrigerator for approximately 12 hours.

Twelve hours later, in a skillet, at high temperature and with a little bit of **vegetable oil**, sauté cubes in order to cook the inside and to brown them slightly on every side (because of cube size, cooking should be relatively quick).

Note that this marinade may also be used for pan-cooked or grilled red meats.

Roasted Chicken

For added flavors (and less toxins), use **organically grown, grain-fed free-range chicken**. Sprinkle generously with the following:

- *Olive oil*
- *Fresh thyme*
- *Fresh rosemary*
- *Freshly crushed coriander seeds*
- *6-7 crushed garlic cloves*

- *Sea salt*
- *Freshly ground black pepper*

Let marinate for 2 hours in the fridge.

Two hours later, in a roasting pan, create a bed of **sliced onions** or **French shallots**, and add a little water so that nothing will stick and burn during subsequent cooking. Set the marinated chicken on this bed, and stuff with **peeled garlic cloves** and fresh thyme. Bake at 400 °F for approximately 1 hour, without covering (calculate approximately 20−25 minutes of cooking time per pound of poultry). Baste chicken occasionally with cooking juices, so it doesn't dry. Finish at broil for a few minutes in order to give it a nice brown color.

Serve with **Market Salad**, or steamed **asparagus** with **vegetable oil**, **sea salt** and **freshly ground black pepper**.

Rosemary & Garlic Roast Leg of Lamb

- *1 leg of lamb*
- *6−8 French shallots*
- *1 bunch of fresh rosemary*
- *1 whole head of garlic cloves*

In a roasting pan, prepare a bed of sliced French shallots and peeled garlic cloves (cut in halves). To prevent burning (during subsequent cooking), add a little water. Set lamb on this bed and brush with **olive oil**; stick fresh rosemary and pieces of garlic cloves (like needles in a pincushion). Add **sea salt** and **freshly ground black pepper** to taste. Also add any remaining rosemary to roasting pan.

Place lamb in oven at 400 °F and roast for 30 minutes, uncovered. Reduce heat to 350 °F and continue to cook for about 1 hour to obtain a *medium-rare result* (30 minutes of cooking time per 2.2 pounds of lamb), which is the recommended preparation for lamb. Baste occasionally with cooking juices so lamb does not dry.

Set for 10−15 minutes on countertop.

When serving, use warmed plates, as lamb tends to cool down very quickly.

Serve with **steamed asparagus**, **green beans** and/or **sautéed mushrooms**.

Seared Salmon Unilateral

On the skin side, cook **fresh salmon fillet** (or other similar fish, like salmon-trout) in a pan at high heat. Searing fish from one side only (unilateral) gets the heat from the pan to slowly cook the fish from the bottom and all the way through. You may reduce heat at one point so the skin doesn't stick and burn. Fish is ready when a <u>thin</u> top layer is warm but still uncooked.

When ready, deposit directly in a serving plate and add:

- *A trickle of olive oil*
- *A dash of freshly squeezed lemon juice*
- *Sea salt*
- *Freshly ground pepper*

You may also add **fresh dill**.

Suggested accompaniments: steamed **asparagus**, **green beans** and/or **Market Salad**.

Shrimps à l'Orange

In a skillet, sweat a few **onions** and add minced **fennel leaves**. Deglaze with **pasteurized orange juice** (be generous...minimum 3-4 cups), and reduce (i.e., make a reduction), leaving enough juice to cook the shrimps.

Next, add **shrimps** and **orange zest** from 1-2 oranges. Shrimps are cooked when pink and opaque (i.e., not translucent anymore).

Add **sea salt** to taste. Serve on a bed of **orange braised fennel** (see Orange & Almond Braised Fennel, but leave out the almonds).

Serve with steamed **asparagus**, **green beans**, **Brussels sprouts**, and/or **sautéed mushrooms**. Pour some of the remaining cooking juices over these accompanying vegetables...mmm, yummy!

Cooking Glossary

Al dente: Italian term, meaning cooked to be firm to the bite; somewhere between hard uncooked and soft very well cooked.

Au gratin: French term, meaning cooked or baked with a topping of either browned breadcrumbs and butter, or grated cheese, or both.

Baste: to moisten (meat or other food) while cooking, with drippings, butter, juices, etc.

Braise: to cook (meat, fish, or vegetables) by simmering slowly in very little liquid.

Bulgur (also bulghur): cracked wheat grains.

Chop: to cut into large pieces (larger than when minced).

Couscous: spherical granules of semolina wheat; also, dish name.

Deglaze: to dissolve the remaining bits of sautéed or roasted food in a pan or pot by adding a liquid and heating, so as to make a sauce incorporating the cooking juices. For most recipes in this book, you will notice that deglazing with freshly squeezed lemon/lime juice requires only 1–2 lemon/lime wedges.

En croûte: French term, meaning food (usually fish, meat or poultry) rolled and covered in herbs and/or spices so that, when baked, a thin crust forms.

Fine-cut: cut into very thin strips.

Grilling: cooking by direct exposure to radiant heat (e.g., over a fire).

Hydrogenated products/spreads: butter-like products made of refined vegetable oils, sometimes blended with animal fats, and emulsified, usually with water or milk; e.g., margarine. Contrary to popular belief, these are not recommended for weight loss.

Infusion: a liquid extract prepared by steeping or soaking (e.g., tea, leaves, root and bark).

Knob: (of butter): approximately a tablespoon amount of butter. A "lump" and a "pat" are terms also used in reference to butter quantity, but are bigger than a "knob".

Mince: to cut into very small pieces (smaller than when chopped).

Organic: refers to methods of growing and processing foods that rely on the Earth's natural resources. Pests and weeds are managed using earth-friendly means such as beneficial insects and mechanical controls, and without use of highly poisonous chemicals. Organic farmers work to build natural nutrients in soil, which help fertilize plants without reliance on synthetic fertilizers. Animals are cared for without any acts of cruelty, and are free to roam around regularly.

Reduce: (or "*to make a reduction*"): to evaporate water from a sauce, a soup or other liquid, usually by boiling.

Roasting: to cook with dry heat, as in an oven or near hot coals.

Sauté: French for a dish of sautéed food. Also, verb (ex. *please sauté these onions*) meaning to cook or brown at high heat in a pan containing a small quantity of butter, oil, or other fat; similar to pan-frying.

Searing: (also pan-searing): cooking food's surface (usually meat, poultry or fish) at high temperature so a caramelized crust forms.

Simmering: to cook in a liquid just below boiling point.

Stir-frying: to cook quickly by cutting into small pieces and stirring constantly in a lightly oiled wok or frying pan, over high heat.

Sweating: (onions): the process of releasing flavors with moisture at low heat. Fat and/or oil, in this case, are used only to hold the non-volatile flavors as they are released from the onions; no browning occurs. In sweating, the onions soften and release their moisture and flavors at a leisurely pace, so they cook in their own juices. *Sautéing* modifies flavors while *sweating* primarily releases flavors already present.

Tabbouleh: commonly, a salad of fine-ground bulgur, parsley, tomatoes, green onions, mint, olive oil and lemon juice.

Tilapia: white-fleshed fish; common name for almost a hundred species of cichlid fishes from the tilapiine cichlid tribe.

Tofu: a soft, bland, white, cheese-like food, high in protein content, made from curdled soybean milk. There are 3 types of tofu:

1. **Soft** - In many cases, soft tofu will be labeled as "silken."
2. **Regular firm** - Also called "medium firm."
3. **Extra firm**

Zest: small pieces of peel, especially thin outer peel, of a citrus fruit, used for flavoring (e.g., *lemon zest).*

Tricks for Eating Out

Eating out at restaurants or at friends is usually a weight-promoting experience. Meals are ill combined, ingredients are processed, and beverages are consumed...tasty maybe, but weight-promoting.

We wish it wasn't so, because eating out is fun, but it is.

The good news is that, with a little determination, it is possible to eat out and still lose weight. It is more complicated because options are fewer, but it is possible. Here are a few tips:

1. When Eating at Friends', It Is Recommended to Let Them Know "Ahead of Time" (As Opposed to "As You Walk Through the Front Door") What You Are and Aren't Willing to Eat.

We are often hesitant to do this because we believe that such a comment will offend them. In our experience, friends (true friends, that is) will appreciate the honesty and will go out of their way to make sure you have a pleasant experience...after all, isn't that what having friends over is all about? Plus, it usually leaves them curious and interested in your new eating habits, maybe even inspired enough to try it themselves.

Be aware, of course, that there are other "friends" who will greet your new eating habits with skepticism and maybe even sarcasm, and this will prove to be unpleasant and discouraging...it'll bc up to you to decide whether or not you want to keep these unsupportive "friends."

2. If You Eat on the Run, Look for Simplicity.

If you eat on the run, say a sandwich while driving or take-out sushi at a computer, then look for ready-meals with *very few* ingredients. As mentioned in Guideline 9 of Step 3, meals tend to get chemically complicated real fast. That's today's reality...we add a little sauce here, a little dressing there...we eat factory-made breads, pastas, muffins, cakes, cookies, soups, etc., all made up of a plethora of ingredients...we consume meals comprised of items from various food groups. In the end, as you now know, this way of eating is very weight-promoting.

Here are a few examples of simplified meals that contribute to weight loss:

- Rice (or eggless noodles) and vegetables, from Asian food take-out places. Although not ideal, you may add soy sauce.

- Roasted chicken or pork from grocery stores' take-out counters. These counters have gotten more popular in the last decade because of the create-your-own-meal possibility, and the availability of items not already part of a combo. Stay away from any fried foods, of course, as these tend to be weight-promoting.

- Sandwiches or subs from a create-your-own sandwich shop. Most common sandwiches are poor combinations (beef, chicken, turkey, ham, seafood, cheese, etc.), so look for the veggie options. The downside of vegetable sandwiches, however, is that they are not usually as tasty as their meat and cheese counterparts. Although not ideal but somewhat tasty, a tomato lettuce sandwich with mayonnaise is an acceptable option. Another option is a vegetarian sub with lettuce, tomatoes, bell peppers, olives, salt and pepper; as for sauce or dressing, a little mayonnaise, mustard, honey Dijon or other sauces (without cheese or nuts) will do. Stay away from add-ons like cheese, and don't have the beverage, chips and cookies usually included in the combo. Have any type of bread except with cheese or nuts.

- Garden burgers (meatless patty) are also a good alternative; if you're really hungry, have 2 or 3 so you won't be tempted to also take fries, soda pop and/or dessert. That's right, having 2-3 garden burgers is better for your weight than having 1 garden burger with fries and a soft drink! Look for patties made with rice and/or oats (starchy), not tofu (protein).

- Ready-to-go salads can be very healthy options. Various vegetable mixes are OK, but be careful with add-ons like chicken, shrimps, eggs, nuts, cheese and dressing. Refer to Step 3 to ensure proper combinations. All-veggie salads (with any type of dressing) are usually the safest bet.

3. Create a New Mindset for the Restaurant "Experience."

As soon as you sit in a restaurant, someone usually comes over and says: "*Something to drink?*" And then, the common course of events will continue with an appetizer, followed by a main course, and finished off by dessert...the whole experience being accompanied by various beverages every step of the way. Break away from this well-established structure! It's OK to be different! Say no to all beverages, make sure that any appetizers and main courses are properly combined, and say no to dessert.

Having the restaurant "experience" be pleasant is mainly a function of your mindset: make it fun and it will be fun...make it complicated, and it will be complicated...simple as that.

4. Take Your Time to Browse the Menu.

As most restaurant menus have a wide selection of weight-promoting items but very few non-weight-promoting ones, it is important to take time and find the options suiting weight loss needs. Here are a few common examples, not all ideal, but all good enough for weight loss:

- Salads. As stated previously, various vegetable mixes are OK, but be careful with add-ons like chicken, shrimps, eggs, nuts, cheese and dressing. Refer to Step 3 to ensure proper combinations. All-veggie salads (with any type of dressing) are still the best option. Tomatoes with bocconcini cheese make a good salad. Cesar salad with bacon bits, no croutons, is also OK. In a goat cheese salad, if the goat cheese is melted on croutons and served on a bed of lettuce, well, just remove the croutons and eat the rest.

- Pasta (preferably eggless), either with vegetables, herbs and olive oil ("pasta primavera") or rosée sauce (do not add parmesan cheese).

- Meat, fowl, fish or seafood with a side of vegetables. Ask that any starchy accompaniments (e.g., bread, rice, pasta or potatoes) be substituted for non-starchy vegetables. Salads are good sides to animal products; adding a little olive oil and balsamic vinegar as salad dressing is acceptable.

- Cheese plates with nuts and tomatoes, no bread, are OK.

- Veggie "sushi" or, for Asian-food connoisseurs, more aptly named kappamaki (cucumber roll) and futomaki (generally vegetarian). Avoid rice and fish/seafood combinations. Also, ask that tamago (eggs) be removed or, if it's already part of the sushi, simply remove it yourself. Soy ("soya") sauce, peanut sauce, ginger or wasabi, although not ideal, are OK.

- If you're in the mood for fish, opt for the sashimi (meaning *"fish only"*). Because fish is protein, do not mix with rice, peanut sauce, fortune cookie, etc. Have just the protein. Unsweetened soy sauce is acceptable.

- Eggplant Parmesan (with melted cheese), not breaded.

5. If Attempting to Properly Combine Your Own Meals, Be Careful with Answers from Your Waiter.

You may be tempted to bring your food combining charts to the restaurant, and end up asking the waiter a wholotta questions about the exact ingredients of every plate to ensure making the right decisions. For example, a pasta dish with vegetables and olive oil on the menu draws your attention and, in order to make sure no ingredients were left out of the menu description, you double check with the waiter to see if it contains any proteins (say meat, cheese or nuts). In our experience, we've noticed that waiters are quick to answer, and very convincingly so, but often, they don't know what they're talking about and you end up with a surprise ingredient in your plate (cheese in pasta dish, or nuts as decoration, for example). It's not the end of the world, of course, for you may simply return the dish and order something else; it just makes things more complicated as you have to wait longer than planned to eat, and may end up not eating at the same time as your dinner companions. Usually, if you tell waiters that you are *deathly allergic* to something, they'll make sure it's not in the dish you've just ordered...

6. In Restaurants, Order from "Sides" or Ask for "On the Side."

Look to the "Sides", "Appetizers" and/or "Starters" parts of the menu. You'll often find easy-to-combine items. In fact, it is possible to make up a whole meal by ordering items only from these menu sections. For breakfast, for example, order 2−3 sides of potatoes, sautéed with onions and herbs...mmm, delicious! Or have 2−3 sides of toasts with peanut butter...or even 3−4 hard-boiled eggs, tomato slices, salt & pepper. OK, OK, it's not your typical "hungry man's" breakfast with eggs and bacon, but what's more important, 20 minutes of eating pleasure and a good 8 hours of tiring digestion, or a sexy shape and a lifetime of satisfaction with your weight? For lunch or dinner, order 2 sides of baked potatoes, with sautéed mushrooms and a garden salad...varied and properly combined!

In addition, when ordering salads or pasta, ask for dressing or sauce "on the side"; this way, you'll be able to ensure that it is well combined before mixing it in all together. Since pasta sauce is usually already mixed-in, double check with the waiter before ordering, thus avoiding an ill-combined meal.

There Are Many More...

To finalize this section, know that these are but a few tricks to eating out. There are many more. As you integrate this new way of eating, you'll find out what works and doesn't work for you. The bottom line is that, although not always simple, eating out is possible, and becomes simpler and easier as you get better with proper food combining.

Case Studies

"It is better to fall short of a high mark than to reach a low one."
— **H. C. Payne, U.S.**
Postmaster General 1902 - 1904

"You cannot plough a field by turning it over in your mind."
— **Unknown**

Because you were introduced to many new concepts throughout the 6 Steps, we included a few case studies so that you may get an idea of what has worked for some of our clients.

As you will see, we have outlined only one *typical* day as it occurred *before* and *after* the individuals read this book; to include *every day* of their weight loss process would have been a little too much.

The *before* part refers to how it was for them just a few weeks prior to their program, whereas the *after* part refers to "after having read" the book and to an average day during their weight loss experience.

You will find the stories of:

- Tracy
- Susan
- Michael

As you go through these case studies, notice the participants' improvement especially on *food combining* and respecting *gastric evacuation time*, and the impact this had on other lifestyle components (exercise, sleep), their weight loss goals and their overall health.

Tracy
(before the program)

Age: 28

Occupation: Media Relations; office job, 40 hours weekly (Mon—Fri, 9—5)

Health: Occasional bouts of eczema and acne, chronic headaches

Height: 5'5   **Weight:** 135 lbs   **Weight loss goal:** 15 lbs

~

Typical workday

7:30 a.m.	breakfast: 1 slice of toast with margarine, yogurt, apple and pasteurized orange juice
9:00 a.m.	at work: coffee with fat-free skim milk and sweetener
12:00 noon	lunch: minestrone soup with soda crackers, tuna salad (with lettuce and light mayonnaise), tomato juice
1:30 p.m.	coffee with fat-free skim milk and sweetener
4:00 p.m.	cheese sticks, low-salt roasted nuts and an apple
5:30 p.m.	at the gym: 20-minute jog on treadmill and 20 minutes of free weights
7:00 p.m.	drinks with friends while munching on a few cheese nachos and chicken wings
9:30 p.m.	back home: a few crackers with low-fat cheese in front of the TV
11:00 p.m.	bedtime: sleep is light, lots of tossing and turning, wakes up for trips to the bathroom or because of a headache (in which case she takes a Tylenol and goes back to bed)

Tracy
(after the book, 3 weeks into her weight loss process)

Health: eczema, acne and chronic headaches have all improved

Weight loss: week 1 = 4 lbs
week 2 = 2 lbs
week 3 = 3 lbs

Total loss after 3 weeks: 9 lbs.
It took her 5 weeks total to reach her goal of 15 lbs

~

Typical workday

7:00 a.m.	1 glass of freshly squeezed orange juice
8:00 a.m.	3 toasts with butter and organic peanut butter
12:00 noon	fried rice with vegetables and a garden salad (with olive oil, salt & pepper)
4:00 p.m.	chocolate candy bar
5:30 p.m.	at the gym: 35-minute jog on treadmill and 20 minutes of free weights
7:00 p.m.	drinks with friends, Cesar salad (no croutons)
9:30 p.m.	back home (no eating)
11:30 p.m.	bedtime: sleep is much better than before (deeper, more recuperative, practically no tossing and turning); average of 1 trip to the bathroom per night; no awakenings due to headaches

Susan
(before the program)

Age: 41

Occupation: Real Estate Agent (high-end clients); works 50-60 hours weekly

Health: circulatory problems in legs (varicosity, water retention), high blood pressure (under medication), diabetes (under medication), chronic migraines, seasonal allergies, chronic lower back pain and insomnia (treated with sleeping pills)

Height: 5'7   **Weight:** 170 lbs   **Weight loss goal:** 40 lbs

---

Typical workday

8:00 a.m.	breakfast: 2 poached eggs, 1 whole wheat toast with margarine, 3 strips of bacon, coffee (with fat-free skim milk and sweetener)
10:00 a.m.	medium-paced walk (30 min.); yoga at home (20 min.)
12:00 noon	business lunch at restaurant: shrimp cocktail, penne with chicken in creamy sauce, glass of white wine, coffee (with fat-free skim milk and sweetener)
3:00 p.m.	muffin & coffee (with fat-free skim milk and sweetener)
6:00 p.m.	ham & cheese sandwich and a diet-soda
9:00 p.m.	back home: fish with rice, glass of wine, sorbet, coffee
10:00 p.m.	recently divorced, Susan now spends time at night on Internet dating sites while sipping a glass of wine
11:00 p.m.	bedtime: sleep is uninterrupted (because of the sleeping pills) and is somewhat recuperative (although Susan always has a feeling of overall numbness the next day)

Susan
(after the book, 9 weeks into her weight loss process)

Health: although some ailments still remain, Susan feels much less   overall discomfort; moreover, her migraines have diminished both in intensity and frequency, her lower back pain has disappeared and her sleep has improved dramatically (no more need for sleeping pills)

Weight loss:

week 1 = 4 lbs	week 4 = 2 lbs	week 7 = 4 lbs
week 2 = 2 lbs	week 5 = 2 lbs	week 8 = 4 lbs
week 3 = 3 lbs	week 6 = 2 lbs	week 9 = 2 lbs

Total loss after 9 weeks: 25 lbs.
It took her 14 weeks to reach her goal of 40 lbs.

―

Typical workday

7:00 a.m.   4 hard-boiled eggs (with salt & pepper), tomato and cucumber slices (also with salt & pepper)

11:00 a.m.   40 minutes of pool aerobics

12:30 p.m.   business lunch at restaurant: Cesar salad (no bacon bits) and penne with rosée sauce

4:30 p.m.   coffee (with cream and sugar)

7:00 p.m.   dinner at home: Seared Salmon Unilateral with a Market Salad

9:30 p.m.   Internet dating session at the computer with her traditional glass of wine

11:30 p.m.   bedtime: as mentioned above, no more need for sleeping pills, sleep is much more peaceful and much more recuperative, energy levels and mental acuity are higher the next day

Michael
(before the program)

Age: 56

Occupation: Security Consultant; semi-retired

Health: pain in knee (arthritis, and he just had knee operation for torn meniscus), chronic heartburn, daily listlessness

Height: 6'4   **Weight:** 308 lbs   **Weight loss goal:** 80 lbs

―

Typical workday

7:30 a.m.	breakfast: pasteurized orange juice, 3 slices of toasts (with jam or cheese), coffee (with powdered creamer and sweetener)
12:00 noon	lunch: chicken club sandwich, fries (with mayo) and a Coke
2:00 p.m.	slow-paced walk (2 hours)
4:00 p.m.	coffee (with cream and sweetener) and 1 muffin
5:00 p.m.	at the gym: 10-minute warm-up on stationary bicycle and 1 hour of free weights (no leg workout because of the knee problem)
8:00 p.m.	back home: beef stew, glass of wine and ice cream
9:00 p.m.	diet soda and glass of Irish Cream
11:30 p.m.	bedtime: non-recuperative sleep, still tired upon awakening and listless (somewhat fatigued) throughout the day

Michael
(after the book, 26 weeks into his weight loss process)

Health: no more discomfort in knee, no more heartburn, improved sleep and better overall energy

Weight loss: After 26 weeks, Michael had lost 66 lbs. He lost an average of 2.7 lbs per week for a total of 30 weeks in order to reach his goal of 80 lbs.

～

Typical workday

7:30 a.m.	breakfast: freshly squeezed orange juice (wait 20 min.), then 2 slices of toast (with butter) and coffee (with cream and sugar)
11:00 a.m.	medium-paced walk (2 hours)
1:00 p.m.	roasted chicken, cherry tomatoes and a glass of water
2:00 p.m.	medium-paced walk (1 hour)
3:00 p.m.	coffee (cream and sweetener)
6:00 p.m.	squash (1 hour)
8:00 p.m.	lettuce, tomato & parmesan cheese salad (with salt, pepper and olive oil) and mineral water
11:30 p.m.	bedtime: calmer, deeper and more recuperative sleep

"One cannot consent to creep when one has an impulse to soar."
– Helen Keller